Keto Diet for Beginners 2020

Joy Cooper

Table of Contents

Introduction

The keto diet has been around for decades, and although the diet plan can be considered controversial there is no arguing its effectiveness for rapid weight loss.

It goes against everything we have learned is the "healthy way of eating." It does not follow the "food pyramid" that everyone was taught in health class and most cardiologists just can't bring themselves to support the diet. Nutritionists and general practitioners are taught that your body needs carbohydrates to fuel your brain. Runners "carb load" before a race to help give them the energy and stamina needed to run long distance. But what if they taught their body to run off of a different type of fuel? What if they could adapt to a different way off eating that would enable them to think more clearly? Give them more energy? And lose weight?

That's what the ketogenic diet can do for you. By eating the Standard Ketogenic Diet of high fat and low carbohydrates you will train your body to run more efficiently and begin to use ketones for energy rather than glycogen. Once you have hit a steady state of ketosis you will begin to see the weight just melt off as your body will be running more efficiently and you will have more energy. Many new keto dieters report weight loss of 10 pounds or more during their first month.

In this book you will learn more about the Ketogenic Diet and where it came from, how it supports weight loss and how to incorporate it into your daily life.

Chapter 1 - How the Ketogenic Diet Works

Before it even had a name, ketogenic diets were being used in the medical world to aide people with neurological disorders. As early as 500 BC fasting was being used as a treatment for epilepsy. In the 1920s physicians began to study how exactly fasting effected the human body and learned that after a period of fasting, the introduction of carbohydrates would cause seizures in epileptic patients, but introducing fat and protein did not. This caused them to look further into the way our bodies processed these different types of food and how they became broken down. They discovered that the body breaks down carbohydrates from our food and converts it to a sugar called glucose. Any excess of this sugar not immediately needed for energy is then stored in the liver and muscles as glycogen. By fasting, their patients were not ingesting any glucose at all for energy so the body had to fall back on its glycogen stores to maintain function of all bodily systems. Once the body ran through all of its glycogen stores it had to find something else to burn for energy, so it began to consume its own fat stores for energy and to keep its brain and organs functioning. The brain is a very hungry organ and requires fuel 24 hours per day, 7 days a week. Because the brain is unable to store fuel it can only run on the glucose or ketones available in the body. If you no longer supply your body with the needed glucose to fuel your brain, out of self preservation, your body will begin to generate ketones to continue to supply your brain. While decades later it is still not fully understood why the body burning fat (ketones) rather than burning glycogen for its energy is so beneficial for cognitive function and neurological disorders, there was no denying the improvements their doctors were seeing in their patients' daily life.   This was the start of the Standard Ketogenic Diet. It did not start out as a means to lose weight but as a means for people suffering to live a better life with less seizures. This diet was used successfully for 40 years as a treatment for epilepsy, especially in children, until the 1st antiepileptic drug was created. Once the new medication became mainstream and the neurologists found that the new drug was working, they decided that remaining on a ketogenic diet or trying to keep their patients on a ketogenic diet takes much more time and discipline than just taking a daily medication, and they began prescribing the new pill. But even today, those seeking a healthier more natural treatment for their ailments and those that have not been able to find a medication that works for them have found that the ketogenic diet can make significant improvements to not only epilepsy but many neurological disorders such as Alzheimer's disease, Parkinson's disease, and chronic migraine, as well as diabetes.

While research is still being done to find out just how much and how the ketogenic diet is able to have such a positive impact on neurological disorders and endocrine diseases, there are many individuals who have found that when their medications fail to fully relieve them of their symptoms, the ketogenic diet can make up much of the difference. It has even been said that a ketogenic lifestyle can help cancer patients. There is no medical research that has been able to fully back up these claims, and most research that has been conducted has been on animals, but the anecdotal evidence is hard to ignore.

While neurologists had been prescribing this way of eating to their patients to ease their neurological distress it was noticed that a natural side effect of this way of eating was weight loss. Even when not counting calories and often eating even more calories than their other patients following a low fat, calorie restricted diet for weight loss, those on a ketogenic diet would lose more weight and at a much faster rate than the other groups. As this information began to make it out to the general public, more and more versions of ketogenic diets were being advertised, but now for weight loss. And everyone was putting their own spin on it. Today, there are many versions of the ketogenic or "keto" diet but what they all have in common are very high in fat, maintain a moderate amount of protein and a very low carbohydrate intake.

So, with so many versions of the diet out there touting their benefits, how do you know which one to follow and which will be the most beneficial to you? Take your time and learn about the diet. Understand, that you will be making great changes to your daily life and health by following this diet. Be sure you are well prepared, and know what foods to eat, which to avoid and how to stay on course when first starting out. You should go into this diet knowing that to reach and maintain long term results you should really think about it as your "new way of life" as opposed to a diet. Diets are short term, once you achieve your desired results you can come off your diet and relax some. If you have been following a ketogenic diet and then feed your body too many carbs, your body will choose the easy burning glucose over converting fat to ketones and you will fall out of ketosis. All is not lost if you do, but it can be difficult to rid yourself of the carb cravings again.

Currently, there are 4 versions of Ketogenic Diets that have become mainstream. Each are best used by different groups of individuals all seeking different results;

There is the Cyclical Ketogenic Diet, or CKD. This version is not recommended for beginners or anyone choosing a ketogenic diet for health concerns such as diabetes or epilepsy. CKD is usually reserved for body builders or athletes, people living a very active lifestyle. While following CKD, these individuals follow the

Standard Ketogenic Diet for 5-6 days per week and 1-2 days they "carb load" while eating very low fat. During their days of "carb loading" these athletes will eat rice, potatoes, pasta, and whole grains, no processed carbs. They are working on filling their muscles with glycogen to enhance their workouts allowing them to perform better and gain muscle growth. Many believe that in order to achieve top performance you must continue to feed your muscles glucose. When feeding your body carbs, it will cause a spike in your insulin levels which will create glycogen to be stored in your muscles. It is known that increased insulin levels will stunt your growth hormone so while you won't gain much in terms of muscle mass during your high carb days you will increase muscle mass during your low carb, high fat days.

In order for a Cyclical Ketogenic Diet to be beneficial you must workout hard after carb loading and incorporate heavy weightlifting to ensure you burn off the glucose to be able to enter back into ketosis again before your next carb loading day. During your carb loading days your carbs are making up about 70% of your diet and about 15% of your calories are coming from protein. The remaining 15% should be made up of healthy fats. During the remainder of the week you would follow something closer to a Standard Keto Diet with Carbs totaling no more than 10% of you daily caloric intake. Due to not staying in a constant state of ketosis this version of the diet would not be beneficial for those looking for weight loss.

Another version of keto for the active person is the Targeted Ketogenic Diet. This method is not as helpful in gaining muscle but may enhance your performance during a workout. This method is most beneficial for those who participate in high intensity interval training HIIT) or cross fit and less so for body builders. TKD is for people who are already fat adapted so they would have already been on a ketogenic diet for awhile and can move in and out of ketosis fairly quickly. This allows you to eat higher amounts of carbs, before, during or after a workout allowing you to improve your workout performance as well as still reaping the benefits a ketogenic diet has to offer, although to a lesser extent.

The targeted version of the ketogenic diet falls between the Standard Ketogenic Diet and the Cyclical Ketogenic Diet and is less beneficial for many dieters. You have to workout hard, doing the correct types of exercise, while eating the right carbs, at the right time and because every individual stores and uses different amounts of glycogen as well as ketones, you don't know how well it will work from person to person. It may take a lot of trial and error and therefore take some time before you see or feel much of any real benefit.

There is also a High Protein version of the ketogenic diet that is designed for those looking to protect their muscle mass such as body builders or older individuals who have to prevent their muscles from breaking down. And while anyone should always consult their doctor prior to starting a new diet plan, this especially goes for those with kidney issues. The increase in protein may be too much on their kidneys when raising their daily intake to about 30% leaving their kidneys unable to filter the way they should and resulting in waste build up in their blood.

Lastly and most common is the Standard Ketogenic Diet. This is the version recommended most to those who are looking to lose weight or help control medical issues such as diabetes or neurological disorders. The SKD is made for people who don't participate in very intense workouts, like yoga or aerobics or even don't exercise at all. It is the Standard Ketogenic Diet that will keep you in a constant state of ketosis allowing you to lose more weight and have increased energy by burning fat 24 hours per day. This is the method, we are going to focus on going forward in this book, starting with how to enter the natural state of ketosis and what exactly it means.

Fat, protein and carbohydrates are your macronutrients or "macros." The most common macro ratio is used in the Standard Keto Diet which consists of 75% fat, 20% protein, and 5% carbohydrates. To get the most benefit out of this way of eating you should think of the 5% carbohydrates as your maximum daily allowance of carbs instead of trying to reach that number.

You will instead want to focus on reaching your fat%. While eating a more standard western diet that is heavy in carbs your body produces its energy from the glucose those carbs have been converted to and any excess is stored as glycogen. By lowering your carb intake and raising the amount of fat you consume so dramatically your body will not have enough glucose to generate the energy it needs and will have to begin burning through your glycogen stores to provide the energy necessary for your daily life. Glycogen is easily burned off by your body and offers fast, easy energy. Unfortunately, because it burns so fast, that energy does not last long and you soon find yourself feeling drained, lacking motivation and hungry again, or looking for a snack to get your focus back. You feed that need with more quick carbs and end up in an infinite cycle where your body is constantly demanding more carbohydrates because you are burning through them too quickly and now find yourself hungry ALL. OF. THE. TIME and still crashing mid day. Once you lower your carbohydrate intake your body will run out of glycogen stores and will have to find a new source of energy. That's where the high fat comes in. Your body also knows how to produce energy from fat but because glucose, and its stored form glycogen burn so easily and fast, it will always be your body's go to when available. It's just not going to work harder than necessary to get the energy it needs for fuel. Because of this, even after following a ketogenic diet strictly for a long time, as soon as you eat any too many carbohydrates, your body will immediately revert back to burning glucose and glycogen for energy. Once your glycogen reserves have been used up, your body will have no choice but to begin to burn fat for energy and your liver will begin to convert that fat into ketones. Like when burning carbs any excess glucose was stored in your body as glycogen, now that your body is burning fat, any excess is now stored as ketones. Once you have enough ketones in your body you reach a natural state of ketosis. While in ketosis our body is able to deliver our energy needs in a more efficient manner that reduces inflammation and offers more energy and clearer thinking.

The Ketogenic Diet not only helps you to lose weight by turning fat into fuel; the high consumption of fat on this diet will also keep you full longer cutting down on your cravings and the need to snack throughout the day. Without trying you will naturally cut calories throughout the day as you eat more satiating foods that will keep your body energized longer so that you will not have that midday slump anymore or need to snack to keep working. Besides weight loss, there are many other benefits that you can reap from a ketogenic diet. One of the many causes of acne is said to be from your blood sugar. Eating a diet that is high in carbs can cause more fluctuations of your blood sugar throughout the day and that can have a negative effect on the health of your skin. By eating healthy fats on the ketogenic diet and reducing carbs you can reduce your overall cholesterol.

Studies have found that your HDL or what is known as your "good" cholesterol levels can increase while simultaneously lowering your LDL or your "bad" cholesterol levels. Following a healthy ketogenic diet has also helped some by aiding their hormone balance and improving their fasting insulin causing a positive effect on endocrine disorders. Many have been able to stop taking medications due to the positive effects of a ketogenic diet. So, while you may have turned to this way of eating just for fast weight loss to be beach ready this summer, you may walk away with many other unexpected benefits. Just remember to always speak with your doctor before starting a new diet plan or making any adjustments to your medications.

So, you know what your macros need to be, how do you track these macros that are so important for reaching and maintaining a state of ketosis? There are quite a few ways to track your macros. You could check the nutrition label on everything before you eat it and track it manually, (which would be very time consuming) or you could use and online nutrition tracker or macro tracker to log your meals into. If you have a smart phone there are multiple apps available in the app stores, both free and paid depending on how much detail you are looking for. Many allow you to just take a picture of the UPC of the food you are looking to log and it enters all of the information for you. The biggest concern is to ensure you are consuming a low amount of carbohydrates. No more than 5% of your macros should consist of carbs and no more that 50 grams, but usually much less, often as low as 20 grams. When calculating carbohydrates for a ketogenic diet you really want to calculate your net carbs. In order to get the amount of net carbs per serving, when checking the nutrition label you subtract the amount of fiber in grams from the amount of carbohydrates in grams and that will give you your net carbs. So, if what you plan to eat has 5 grams of carbs and 3 grams of fiber, that item only contains 2 grams of net carbs. Once you become comfortable with the diet you may find that you no longer have the need to track your food so diligently as you fall into a routine and enjoy eating the same foods often or are able to estimate the macronutrients more accurately, but you should wait at least 3 months before you think about no longer tracking your macros. It can take a while to get used to actual portion sizes and many foods can vary greatly between brands.

When it comes to meal options, some find that trying to make keto friendly versions of their favorite foods helps them to stay on track and cut back on the feeling of being deprived. It can also provide more of a variety of foods if you are the type to get bored easily when eating the same foods every day. Others find it easier and more cost efficient to stick to whole foods with minimal processing and ingredients. Basic meats and a side of vegetables works for them and they don't spend much time on involved recipes or sauces. After a while, many even naturally cut back on the seasonings in preference of allowing the taste of the food shine through. Whichever you find works best in your life is the way you should go. Remember, while there are some basic "rules" to follow, this is your journey to weight loss and a healthier life, you choose the path.

Chapter 2 - Adaptation

There's more to adaptation that just your body switching from glucose to ketone usage for fuel. Your body will be going through many changes and some of them you will notice by the way you are feeling. There is no doubt that once you have become fully fat adapted you will be able to reap all of the great many benefits of keto such as weight loss and increased energy. But before you can become a fat burning machine, we need to get into the part that no one talks about. Adaptation. After so many years of your body taking the easy way out and relying on the easily converted, fast burning glucose for energy it is going to take some time for your body to become accustomed to the slower burning and more efficient ketones for fuel. Because no one ever talks about adaptation and only ever wants to share the positive side of the diet, it is during this time that many people think something must be wrong. They must be getting sick, or this diet just doesn't work for them and they give up. Just days before their body has had the chance to acclimate to all of the changes they have made, they throw in the towel and reach for the comfort of those carbs, losing out on all of the benefits.

While the adaptation phase is not fun to go through, once you come out the other side you will be a new person. So many jump into this diet not knowing what to expect, but if you go into this way of eating well prepared and aware that everyone goes through an adaptation phase and what that can look like, your results will be more positive. Keep reading so that you will know what the symptoms are, and how you may feel as your body starts to run out of glycogen stores and begins to go after the fat you want it to burn away, and don't let it scare you off. You can get through it as long as you know what's coming. It isn't harmful or dangerous, it doesn't mean this diet wasn't meant for you, and it will be over soon.

The human metabolism is incredibly flexible when it comes to fuel. Cultures throughout history all over the world have adapted to subsist on what is available to them leaving some with 80% of their energy coming from carbohydrates and others with 80% of their energy from fats. This adaptation by culture has evolved slowly over time, through many generations. While for our ancestors it was caused by necessity due to the climate in their area and the availability of foods. We now have a choice of what foods to eat. When we decide to begin a ketogenic diet, the majority of us coming from a carb heavy lifestyle from which we were brought up in, to very little carbs in a very short period of time, we should expect an adjustment period. Some notice the changes almost immediately, within a matter of days, while it may take a couple of weeks before others begin to see or feel the difference, but just about everyone goes through some sort of period of adaptation. Carbs are sugar, and sugar is known to be addictive. Your body has grown accustomed to generating energy from carbs, it's easy, it's familiar, now that you are no longer supplying your body with this form of fuel it must find a new method to keep itself running. That's where the high fat comes in. As your body learns to break down the fat and create ketones to fuel you, you will find it is working much harder (at least at first) than it did to break down carbs to run off of their sugar for energy. But the energy created from ketones is much more efficient, and burns slower keeping you satisfied longer and providing your body and mind with many benefits. But before you can get there, this extra work of burning off the fat as ketones, this can cause what is known as the "keto flu."

Don't worry though. You will not have to go through several months of adaptation to benefit from this diet. Most of the time your body is adapting you will not even notice it, except during the initial period of the adaptation phase, also known as the keto flu because it share many symptoms in common with the actual flu. In the early stages of ketosis the keto flu can have many symptoms and it will effect each individual differently. Some people begin to notice the symptoms just 3 days to a week into their new way of eating while others may not be affected until 2 weeks to almost a month after starting the diet. The most common symptoms reported are fatigue, nausea, vomiting, headache, irritability, weakness, muscle cramps, dizziness, poor concentration, difficulty sleeping, sugar cravings and digestive discomfort. I know it sounds like a lot, but most people do not get all of the symptoms and usually not all at once. Expect to at least have the digestive discomfort. Adding that high amount of fat takes some time to adjust to. Symptoms usually last a few days to 2 weeks but some have been reported them to last up to a month and they have caused many people to give up on this diet. There is no need to give up, there are ways to reduce your discomfort to get you through this adaptation phase and once you do, you will see the benefits of this way of eating in your increased energy, cognitive clarity and narrowing, leaner waist.

Now, it is still not fully understood whether fat or carbs are better for your body in the long run. Or how long it would take for your body to truly optimize ketone use and that is because there haven't been any long term studies on how a long term high fat, low carb diet would effect a person. Although it has been proven that you are not fully fat adapted or in an optimal state of ketosis just because you have ketones in your blood, most scientists studying nutrition have felt they would be able to get adequate results on how high fat will affect the many systems of the body within just a couple of weeks. While still being researched, it has been found that you may be in a state of nutritional ketosis in as little as 3 days but there are multiple other complex changes going on in your body all at the same time, and some will take longer than others. Your body is generating ketones to feed the brain, heart and muscles. Your tissue is adapting to allow more ketone use by the brain, and a reduction of Reactive Oxygen Species (ROS) production causing less tissue damage. It is not until your body and all systems have fully adapted to the changes that we will really be able to see how you will be affected long term and it often can take weeks to even several months to fully recover from the adaptation phase of this diet change to be able to recognize the amount of benefits you have received. What has been researched is the difference in weight and fat loss people see when on a ketogenic diet versus a more typical calorie restricted diet. Studies have shown that the ketogenic diet always shows increased numbers in weight lost in less amount of time.

So, how do you know that you are in ketosis? There are a few ways; you could go out to your local pharmacy and purchase ketone strips or a monitor to test the level of ketones present in your blood or urine, but you can also tell by some of the changes you will notice in your body. Some side effects of ketosis that you may notice are frequent urination or bad breath, often smelling of acetone (which is the smallest ketone), rapid weight loss, (I know, finally a side effect you were hoping for!) and decreased appetite.

There are ways to combat the negative symptoms of adaptation until your body adjusts:

Frequent urination-

It is known that glycogen is used to store energy in the body while using carbohydrates for fuel. Each glycogen molecule is bound to a few grams of water so as your body burns through your glycogen stores it will release a lot of water causing the frequent urination. This is often a time when you will see weight drop by significant amounts almost overnight. That's why it is always said that you are mostly just losing water weight at the beginning of a diet.

<u>Headaches</u>

The frequent urination also can lead to dehydration and electrolyte imbalance causing the constipation, headaches and dizziness. Remember to drink plenty of water to fight off the dehydration, and try adding salt to your food. Pink Himalayan salt is great for the added minerals. Adding potassium rich, green leafy vegetables to your diet can help as well as drinking a cup of bullion. While this will not help the frequent urination remember that it is helping your body to adapt and become a more efficient fat burning machine and once it does (usually in a couple of weeks) you will see a decrease in your need to urinate as well as your headaches.

<u>Bad breath</u>

Often called keto breath it is compared to nail polish remover and is caused by the increased levels of acetone (a type of ketone) in your bloodstream. This will usually go away on its own within a few weeks. If this symptom is troublesome for you or makes you feel self conscious, drink plenty of water and use some sugar free breath fresheners to help keep your breath fresh.

<u>Fatigue</u>

This is one of the symptoms that causes people to quit just before they have adapted. Fatigue is different than just being sleepy. It is a state of mental and/or physical exhaustion. It's recommended that you get lots of rest during your first 4-6 weeks of a ketogenic diet. It is usually best not to exercise during the beginning of this diet and just allow your body to get used to running on ketones. Once your body has adapted you will notice an increase in your energy levels and starting or returning to an exercise routine would be more possible.

<u>Digestive Discomfort</u>

Unfortunately, there is not a whole lot you can do about this one except to ride it out. Your body will get used to the higher amounts of fat and if you are having problems with diarrhea or loose stools, it will go away with adaptation. If you have been struck with constipation it is again usually caused by dehydration and the amounts of water being released by your body. Increasing your water intake can help with this one too.

<u>Muscle Cramps and Dizziness</u>

These symptoms are most often caused by dehydration and electrolyte imbalance as well. Continue to drink plenty of water, add salt and potassium to your diet and get plenty of rest.

Another option that may be able to help you while in the adaptation phase is adding more fat to your diet. Chances are you still are not eating enough and you are not correctly calculating the amount of fat in your foods or are not tracking it at all. Increasing your fat intake will encourage your body to go into ketosis faster, enabling you to get over your flu even sooner. To add fat to your diet quickly you could add coconut oil to your meals. Coconut oil contains MCTs which we will go over in an bit more detail later. These MCTs are a fat that is easy for your body to breakdown and use right away. You can also purchase and MCT oil supplement rather than adding coconut oil.

While everyone will experience adaptation to ketosis differently with their symptoms ranging from mild to severe, everyone can get through the adaptation process and by maintaining the ketogenic diet and staying in a permanent state of ketosis you won't have to go through it again and can reap the many benefits ketosis provides. The majority of your flu symptoms can be lessened by staying hydrated, getting enough rest and adding salt to your diet. So, drink, drink, drink and get some rest. Soon enough you will be feeling great!

Now, many confuse ketosis and ketoacidosis which causes much of the keto diet's bad reputation. Nutritional ketosis occurs once the body starts to burn fat for energy, while ketoacidosis is a possibly life threatening condition that occurs when the body thinks it is starving and begins to break down fat and protein too quickly. While ketoacidosis usually only affects diabetics it can, in rare circumstances, affect others as well. If a person does not have enough insulin, their body is unable to move glucose from the blood into cells where it is needed for energy. This causes dangerous levels of glucose and ketones to accumulate in the blood.

Symptoms of ketoacidosis would include many of the same symptoms as the keto flu such as thirst, frequent urination, and fatigue. But also may include high blood glucose levels, increasing levels of ketones in their urine and dry or flushed skin. As it progresses, worsening symptoms may include nausea, stomach pain, vomiting, difficulty breathing, a fruity odor in their breath as well as confusion and loss of consciousness.

If you think there is a chance that you are in a state of ketoacidosis or are more susceptible, a doctor can test either your blood or urine to determine whether or not a person is in ketosis or ketoacidosis. While ketoacidosis is a medical emergency that can progress rapidly it is also treatable typically by hospital admission with insulin therapy and electrolytes.

If you have diabetes and are planning to follow a ketogenic diet, you can reduce your risk by monitoring your blood glucose levels and testing your urine for ketones if your blood glucose is over 240mg/dl. You could also avoid exercise if blood glucose levels are high and take your insulin as prescribed.

So, now that you are armed with the knowledge and tools to get through your period of adaptation, don't fret. We've all had to get through a couple of days of work or school not feeling 100%, but never before have we known that once we make it out the other side of this flu, we are going to feel amazing and will finally be burning fat all day every day. Just a few days (ok, sometimes a week or so) of feeling down and uncomfortable will be worth all that you will be gaining once in nutritional ketosis. But before you get started on your ketogenic diet, take a little bit of time to learn some more about ways to increase your fat burning while enjoying extra free time and little to no added effort.

Chapter 3 - Intermittent Fasting and OMAD

Fasting has been going on for thousands of years, for many different reasons and across many different religions and cultures. Presently, fasting is being used in new forms as a way to increase weight loss and improve health. It is believed that fasting is a non stressful way to decrease your calorie intake while still eating all of the foods you enjoy. You now just enjoy them for limited times during the day or week.

One of the many ways to aide you in your weight loss journey is intermittent fasting or IF. Some try intermittent fasting as a way to lose weight by itself with mixed results. When using IF with a Standard American Diet it can often cause weight gain due to carb cravings and increased calorie intake during meal periods. But, it is known that fasting is one of the quickest ways of getting your body into ketosis, after all, it is how the ketogenic diet was founded, so combining fasting with a ketogenic diet can only help you burn more fat. Think about it. If your body has become fat adapted and burns off the fat you are consuming for energy, the only place it can turn to when in a fasted state to produce energy is your stored fat. So, while fasting, your body is just going through your fat stores making you leaner while you go about your day. (and even while you sleep.)

Intermittent fasting is a term used for fasting for a predetermined amount of time and then allowing yourself to eat in the remaining time window during a 24 hour period. There are again, many different methods of intermittent fasting, each having their own list of pros and cons. Some methods can be dangerous and unhealthy for individuals not already fat adapted or used to fasting. Intermittent fasting does not dictate what foods the dieter should eat but instead dictates when it can be eaten. Intermittent fasting is most often used for diet and weight loss but some use it trying to mimic the way our hunter-gatherer ancestors would have eaten. Since they did not have food available to them at the ready they often ended up in a state of fasting while sleeping, then going out to hunt and prepare their meat prior to being able to eat it. At times even having to fast for days.

One method of fasting is known as the EAT-STOP-EAT method. This involves eating normally most days but then fasting for a full 24 hours once or twice each week.

The 5:2 method is somewhat similar to the EAT-STOP-EAT method. Followers of this fasting plan eat normally 5 days each week and then eat no more than 500 calories on the other 2 non consecutive days.

These two methods of intermittent fasting rely on calorie restriction over the week to create a caloric deficit that should lead to weight loss. For many people, these methods do not work for many reasons, but mostly because they are difficult to follow faithfully. Not eating anything for a full 24 hour period is very difficult and should only be attempted by those who are used to fasting for long periods of time. It may cause you to feel faint or dizzy, some even feel confusion and weakness. But also, many people find that they actually overeat during their meal periods because they have become so hungry during their fast they end up eating too quickly when they do eat and end up consuming even more calories than they would had they not fasted at all.

Lastly, the most commonly used method of intermittent fasting and the best option for those new to fasting, is the 16/8 method. This method involves fasting for 16 hours a day and only allowing yourself to eat for the remaining 8 hours of the day. This is one of the only methods that is considered safe enough for long term, everyday use. During this period of fasting since you are not consuming any food for your body to turn into ketones (or even glucose) your body must rely on its fat stores for energy. By having to use the fat stored in your body rather than what would be readily available in the food you consume it is enabling you to move the needle on the scale much faster. Even when you are sleeping your body has to keep producing energy to allow for brain functions, organs running, blood pumping and even just to breathe. These basic needs all take energy from the body and it has to come from somewhere. Might as well come from the unneeded fat you have stored away!

If interested in intermittent fasting and wondering how to get started on the 16/8 method of IF you should first take a look at what your daily life is like. Do you work days? Nights? Do you HAVE to eat breakfast to wake up and get moving in the morning? Do you like to entertain or go out to dinner with friends? These questions would all be important to consider prior to making a decision on when your 8 hour time frame for eating should be. Many choose to skip breakfast and allow themselves to eat between noon and 8pm. This allows them to fast overnight while sleeping so their body burns off all of the fat they ate that night and begins burning through their stored fat into the morning at work or school allowing time for lunch and dinner and then to start burning all over again. This time frame is especially beneficial for those who enjoy dinner with friends often. Others MUST have breakfast to wake up in the morning and start their day. If this sounds like you, choosing a timeframe of 8am-4pm then fasting the remaining 16 hours may work better for your lifestyle. You'll burn through the fat you've eaten during the day while you are working and running errands and start burning through your fat stores as you go to bed. Whatever timeframe you do choose remember that you do not have to "make up" for those lost hours of eating, nor do you have to eat during the entire 8 hours. Intermittent fasting should allow you to cut down on the amount of food you take in naturally and help you to burn more fat during your fasting period. As always, you should listen you your body and stop eating when you are no longer hungry. Do not allow yourself to make the mistake of overeating and adding unnecessary calories to your diet.

When first starting IF you may find that you are hungry outside of the 8 hour time frame that you have decided will be your window to eat. Giving yourself some time to adjust and choosing the right foods to eat will help you stay satiated longer. Also, be sure to stay hydrated during your fasting periods. Drinking plenty of water, coffee, teas or any other calorie free, unsweetened beverages may help you to feel less hungry and get you through another hour. If after a week or so, you do find that you have chosen the wrong time frame for your meal periods, make the appropriate adjustments and continue on with your fasting cycle. This is still your journey. Make it work for you.

Many people find it easiest to start the 16/8 method by not eating anything after dinner then skipping breakfast. Depending on your dinner time, for most this would bring them to fasting for about the 16 hours they are working towards. To help keep you from snacking after dinner have a warm tea to help you relax, or many find it helpful to brush their teeth right away after dinner (or even when that snack craving hits), the mint flavor of the toothpaste will often keep you from wanting to eat anything else and it helps to signal to your brain that you are done eating for the night. Or just go to bed and get some much needed rest. By the time you wake up you will have already fasted for 12 hours! Now skip breakfast if you can or delay it a bit to a more convenient time if you find yourself rushing around in the morning to get kids off to school or get ready for work. If you cannot hold off for the full 16 hours to start, try delaying your first meal by an hour each day until you reach you fasting goal. Try to cut out snacks between meals and you will soon find it's easy to fast for 16 hours and won't even notice you are skipping breakfast and are still not yet hungry when lunch time rolls around.

While keto does allow snacks like nuts or cheese crisps, these foods will not take much time for your body to burn through. So, if choosing to fast focus on eating a real, whole meal that includes a high fat meat such as a rib eye steak with a side of broccoli or asparagus or even eggs cooked in butter with a side of bacon. You can even have both, you have a full 8 hours! These complete meals will keep you more satisfied and cut down on your cravings during your fasting periods. Soon, you will find that you are not so hungry as often. And that's ok. The foods you are eating now are more nutrient dense than the carbs you were burning through before. Just pay attention to the signals your body is giving you. There is no need to force yourself to eat when you are not hungry.

When eating complete, high fat meals during your 8 hours of "meal time", you may find as you become more comfortable with the diet and have become better adjusted to the higher fat foods and you are not hungry as often. You may find that you have fallen into a routine where you are only eating One Meal A Day or OMAD. This is a method that many people choose, and others fall into it naturally. It is just another form of intermittent fasting. While there is no need to strive to reach this point, it is perfectly normal and you should not force yourself to eat just because you have always been told to eat 3 meals a day, or many small meals throughout the day. Much of what you have learned about metabolism just isn't true. You will not gain weight just because you skipped breakfast, the same goes for eating breakfast. Just because you eat breakfast every morning does not mean it will boost your metabolism and cause you to lose weight.

You do not need to eat many small meals each day to increase your metabolism and retain muscle. Remember, food is fuel and should be used as such. While your body can store away excess fat as ketones, it is not necessary or recommended to overeat. You must be mindful when using any form of intermittent fasting as it can easily cause you to eat more than you normally would for fear of being hungry later so you overstuff yourself during meal times. It will help if you eat slowly and pay attention to your meal instead of zoning out in front of the tv. Sit down at the table with family and friends and eat foods you enjoy. Catch up on everyone's day and take your time. When you begin to feel full, stop eating. Don't wait until you have overeaten and are too stuffed to move. This will also help you to gain a more positive, healthy relationship with your food that does not involve just eating out of habit or boredom and may find that you have much more free time during the day.

While you most likely have already learned for yourself, that intermittent fasting can be convenient, and a time saver, you may wonder what is happening to your body during these fasting periods? And, is it safe? It has been found that your insulin levels will be lower allowing your body to access your stored fat easier to enable weight loss. Your body will also work on repairing its cells. During intermittent fasting your body will begin a process called autophagy which will allow it to remove protein build up and damaged or dead cells. Fasting may also change how your body develops certain conditions and diseases. It can even lower your risk of type 2 diabetes and reduce inflammation. Some studies have even found that intermittent fast may be able to extend longevity.

While studies so far have only been on animals, several have found that fasting has a very positive effect on brain health. One study showed that practicing intermittent fasting improves both the brain's functions as well as the brain's structures, while other studies have shown that fasting could increase the generation of nerve cells that will help to enhance cognitive function. It has also been shown to help relieve inflammation which can help prevent neurodegenerative disorders such as Parkinson's and Alzheimer's diseases. Though still lacking in human studies, the research that has been done has shown many positive side effects and benefits for a something that take little effort to initiate and follow.

Intermittent fasting isn't for everyone though. As mentioned previously, IF may cause some people to actually increase the amount of food they eat, while trying to make up for the hours they were fasting. This too may lead to digestive problems and an unhealthy relationship with food. If you have been diagnosed with an eating disorder, IF may not be right for you and as always speak to your doctor about your plans to start a method of intermittent fasting before going forward with it. Start slowly if you need to, gradually decreasing the amount of hours you are eating and increasing the hours you are fasting until you reach your desired ratio of 16/8. If you feel sick or have health concerns, stop the fasting and talk with a trusted medical professional.

With so many benefits, it's worth giving it a try along with your ketogenic diet. You may not want to make so many changes all at once though. Maybe allow yourself to become fat adapted first. Get comfortable with the diet and foods available and after a month or so of keto when you have begun to make it a habit and you are starting to feel less of an appetite, begin intermittent fasting. The 16/8 method is easy and many unknowingly, are already fasting even if not everyday, just when they skip a meal, whether due to time constraints or lack of hunger. It can only benefit you and help you attain your weight loss goals faster with little to no change of the foods you have already been eating on the ketogenic diet.

Chapter 4 - Ketogenic Food and Supplements

There are many paths on a ketogenic diet. Some choose to try to make their favorite dishes "keto friendly", others choose to keep it simple and stick to whole food options only. Many find themselves evolving over time to more simple food options and recipes. Choose whichever path will enable you to follow this way of eating and enjoy it. Remember it can take 4-6 weeks to get through adaptation and about 90 days before you will begin to recognize all of the benefits of this diet. Give it an adequate amount of time and don't give up because you think it is too complicated, or expensive. This diet doesn't have to cost any more than what your are eating now and once in ketosis you will find you can save quite a bit on your grocery shopping now that you are not hungry all of the time and even more if you are combining it with intermittent fasting.

The ketogenic diet is so popular because you see fast weight loss results, but also because you don't have to feel deprived. You are not counting calories and restricting portion sizes and you have more choices of food than in many other diets. The only restriction when following a ketogenic diet is no sugar and low carb. Your carb intake should be no more than 50 grams and often a lot less than that depending on your calorie consumption. Remember potatoes and corn and all starchy foods will just break down to glucose too. So, fill your plate with low carb, high fat, healthy foods such as meats and seafood. Cut out the carb heavy starches and don't forget to eat plenty of healthy fats too.

Most diets instruct you to eat lean meats with lots of fruits and vegetables and to watch your calorie intake, the ketogenic diet is not like that and that's one of the reasons why it is so popular. While other diets are telling you to fill your plates with fruits and salads and to maybe add a little lean protein those living the keto life are enjoying plates of steak and onions covered in cheese sauce with sides of asparagus and avocado and even desserts. The ketogenic diet flips other diets on their heads and only those brave enough to try something "new" and different from all of the other diets out there will see all of the greatness this diet has to offer. I know it seems impossible that eating such a high amount of fat could possibly cause you to lose so much weight. But that's the great thing about ketosis, the more fat you eat the deeper into ketosis, you will go. Now, there is little to no benefit of being in a deeper state of ketosis so no need to go overboard and live on deep fried butter, just know that this diet works and you will feel great. So, no need to feel hungry and don't delay anymore. You don't have to "wait until Monday", or wait until "after the holidays" start now, and still enjoy your favorite foods.

Please see the below chart for just some of the Keto approved foods.

Meat	Seafood
Beef	Calamari
Chicken	Anchovies
Duck	Haddock
Lamb	Hake
Pork	Mackerel
Turkey	Prawns
Bacon (Look for the lowest amount of sugar possible.)	Mussels
	Sardines
Sausages (Watch out for fillers, gluten and sugars.)	Salmon
	Squid
Eggs	Tuna
(You can eat all parts of the animal and are encouraged not to trim the fat and enjoy the skin.)	Trout
	Scallops
Vegetables	**Fats**
Asparagus	All animal fats
Artichokes	Avocado Oil

Green beans	Butter
Cucumber	Coconut Cream/Milk
Broccoli	Coconut Oil
Cabbage	Beef Tallow
Brussel Sprouts	Extra Virgin Olive Oil
Kale	Ghee
Cauliflower	Lard
Lettuce	Heavy Cream
Mushrooms	Macadamia Nut Oil
Peppers	Mayonnaise (Homemade)
Radishes	
Olives	
Pumpkin	
Onion	
Spinach	
Tomatoes	
(Most veggies that grow above ground are safe. Any root vegetables that grow underground are usually too starchy and high in carbs.)	
Flours	**Fruits**
Almond Flour	Berries
Hazelnut Flour	Coconut
Coconut Flour	

Other Nut Flours	(Fruit is very high in natural sugar, be very careful and eat sparingly)
Drinks Water Sparkling water Any and all teas (No milk) Coffee (With butter or cream no milk)	**Sugar Substitute** Erythritol Xylitol Stevia
Seeds Sunflower Seeds Flax Seeds Chia Seeds Pumpkin Seeds	**Nuts** Almonds Macadamias Pecans Hazelnuts Brazils Walnuts Pinenuts
Dairy Butter Cream Feta Cheese Blue Cheese Parmesan Cheese Cream Cheese Ghee	**If you find yourself at a stall or having difficulty losing weight, cutting back on the nuts and dairy will often help.**

| Greek Yogurt
(Any dairy you eat should always be full fat. You may also include other high fat cheeses.) | |

This is not an all inclusive list and as you can see there is no reason to ever feel deprived on this diet. Any oily fish would be a great addition, game, high fat cheeses, this is just a basic list to get you started. With keto, you can still eat full meals and even desserts. But there are some foods that you will want to be careful with, they may be easy to eat too much of or have hidden ingredients you may not expect. When you get started on this way of eating you will find there is often a great difference in carb count just from brand to brand due to the ingredients used. So, when starting out, read all labels until you know which brands you can trust, and which brands will best fit in your new healthy lifestyle.

So, when you are out doing your grocery shopping be sure to look out for these tricky foods:

Bacon-Everyone loves bacon! You don't have to give up bacon for weight loss or even substitute it with turkey bacon. It can even be made ahead of time and kept in the fridge for when you need a quick snack. Just remember to look for bacon without nitrites or nitrates and with the least amount of sugar (carbs) possible. The majority of the carb count in bacon is from the sugar used in the curing process. It will be difficult but not impossible to find bacon with little to no sugar so just remember to steer clear of the flavored (think brown sugar) bacon and read the ingredient and nutrition facts before purchasing. Bacon can be great to help you hit your fat %, just don't overdue it, that sugar can add up too.

Fruit-I know! You have always been told fruit is healthy and you should eat multiple servings per day. Not on the ketogenic diet. Most fruits are high in sugar, it may be a natural sugar but it is still enough to throw you out of ketosis. Small amounts of berries are usually safe but no other fruits should be eaten in any form.

Dairy-While dairy is acceptable on a keto diet, and heavy cream and cream cheese can be great for the added fat, it can often hinder weight loss. Dairy can be a very calorie rich food and the carbs add up quickly. A glass of milk will have an average of 10 grams of carbs. Dairy products have also been known to round down their carb counts, so while the nutrition label may state 0 grams per serving, it may be closer to .7 grams which will add up throughout the day. Anything you do have that is dairy, (think cheeses, not milk) remember to choose the full fat version, no need for low fat cheeses in this way of eating.

Vegetables-Another one of those "healthy" food groups. The easiest way to remember if it is acceptable is whether it grows above or below ground. Most vegetables that grow below ground are high in starch and high in carbohydrates which all means sugar or glucose to our bodies. Stick to veggies that grow above ground like broccoli, cabbage, spinach, and asparagus. They still have carbs but in much lower amounts so it can be difficult to overdue it on the leafy greens. Bell peppers, onions, and tomatoes (I know, they're really a fruit) are a bit higher in carbs and can add up quickly if you use a lot in a dish so be careful and use your macro tracker when planning your meals out.

Nuts-Nuts are a great snack, both a great source of fat and protein, especially macadamias, but can average 3 grams of carbs per serving and they are WAY too easy to overeat! The serving size is usually much smaller than you would expect. Check your nutrition facts and be careful. They are great to enjoy in moderation or as a crunchy topping to a salad or dessert.

Condiments can be a bit tricky at times on a ketogenic diet as well. But don't worry. You don't have to eat all of your foods dry. Regular yellow mustard, stone ground or even most French Dijon mustards are all sugar free and carb free. Just be sure not to use the honey mustards as they all contain sugar. With only 1 gram of carbs per serving, soy sauce can make a great addition to you meal. Hot sauce is a staple in the low carb, keto world. With 0 grams of sugar and 0 grams of carbs, you really can put it on anything. Many salad dressings are keto-friendly but you will have to read the labels as they can vary quite a bit brand to brand, but you can usually find some safe full fat versions of ranch, Caesar, Italian and blue cheese salad dressings that you can use as a salad topping or even as a marinade for your meats. There are also sugar free and no sugar added ketchups and barbecue sauces. Make sure you read the label. No sugar added does not necessarily mean there is no sugar. Make sure it will work within your macro plan. And of course, Mayonnaise. While there are now many different types of mayo available in the grocery stores using many different types of oils, it may just be safer to make your own.

For an easy homemade mayo recipe that actually tastes store bought you will need:

2 cold, large eggs

1 teaspoon of yellow mustard

2 Tablespoons of fresh lemon juice (this will act as a preservative)

½ teaspoon of pink Himalayan salt

1 cup of sesame oil

½ cup of grapeseed oil (you can use all sesame oil if you choose)

Blend all ingredients except for the oils in a blender or food processor until well combined.

With the blender still running, slowly pour your oils into the mix. You want to take at least a minute to pour the oils in to the egg mixture.

Once the oils have been added, check your mayonnaise for consistency. If you find that it can use some adjusting, add more oil in one Tablespoon at a time while the blender is running until desired consistency is reached.

Recipe makes about 2 cups of mayonnaise. Store the mayo in a glass jar in the refrigerator for up to 5 weeks.

You will also find that because keto has become so popular, there are many companies marketing supplements, snacks and heat and serve meals. The most commonly used supplement being MCT oil. MCT stands for medium chain triglyceride. This oil is made up from medium-length chains of fats (triglycerides) which are easily digested. They are thought to help keep you in a state of ketosis as well as to help keep you feeling full longer. While these supplements are not needed on a ketogenic diet, they may help you burn more fat and reach ketosis faster. But there really hasn't been enough research done on them and with so many companies looking to make money fast be sure to do your homework on them before trying them out.

Another supplement that's available commercially are exogeneous ketones. These are a class of ketones that can be ingested in pill or powder form to mix with a liquid. Using the ketone supplement may help you to reach a nutritional state of ketosis faster and help you to maintain the state easier, it can provide you with an instant supply of ketones even if your body is not in a state of ketosis before you have taken them. There are a couple of different types of supplemental ketones and many companies offering them. Commercially available supplements would include ketone salts and ketone esters each having their own effects on the body and blood, some are slow burning for lasting energy and decreased hunger while others will burn quickly. They all will enable your body to use less glucose.

Some manufacturers advertise using their supplements to attain a state of nutritional ketosis and lose weight without decreasing the carbs in your diet. While you will have more ketones in your blood and you will test in ketosis, studies have found that the body will still use fewer ketones as fuel due to the ready available glucose from the carbs which will negatively effect your weight loss. Exogenous ketones can be beneficial at the start of a ketogenic diet to help you reach a nutritional state of ketosis faster, but if you continue to eat large amounts of carbs while taking them they will inhibit your weight loss. Because you will be providing your body with ketones, it will be making little to none of it's own ketones so it will not be burning as much fat as it would normally, just the ketones and glucose you are supplying your body with. Also, you will have to take the supplement multiple times a day which can become very expensive. If you plan to supplement with exogenous ketones, it would be best to only use them during your first week of the ketogenic diet and be sure to reduce your carbs appropriately. Otherwise, you may derail your own efforts at weight loss.

There are already a ton of snack bars available on the market and it seems like they are coming out with more and more everyday. Heat and serve meals are also available in many grocery stores advertising the convenience of their quick and easy meal but they are often higher in carbs than "real" food options that you could make yourself with larger portion sizes that would keep you satiated longer. If you're on the go and have to eat something "right now", a keto snack bar won't hurt as long as it doesn't become a habit. But making these snack bar your "go to" can slow down your weight loss. These snack bars and meals are high in calories and have many processed ingredients and chemicals. Whenever possible, stick to minimally processed or organic foods. Consuming natural foods are more nutritionally beneficially and naturally lower in calories. Limiting the amount of chemicals you are ingesting will help reduce inflammation and digestive discomfort.

Like any diet, you will get out of it what you put into it. You could fall into a state of nutritional ketosis by eating just bacon and butter or even just the processed snack bars and frozen meals. But eating this way will not give you all of the vast nutrition that following a healthy unprocessed ketogenic diet will. By consuming meats and green salads with healthy fats like avocado or olive oil you will feel the difference by providing your body with a more diverse bouquet of vitamins and nutrients overall. What makes this diet fun and easy to follow is the options it gives you in food. Of course it would be ok to indulge sometimes on an a delicious dessert or keto "candy bar" or relax and just heat up a frozen meal on particularly long and tiring day, but it will be better for your body and your waistline if you don't make a habit of it.

Chapter 5 - Keto Meal Ideas

Keto meals can be as simple or as complicated as you would like and can fit all budgets. While a ribeye might have the perfect fat to protein ratio, it can get a bit pricey if eating it every night. Ground beef and chicken thighs are some great options to add into your meal planning and will help you save too!

This diet can be VERY different from the way some are used to eating. Many households live on meat and starches daily with some added bread and snacks. Some rarely eat fresh veggies or salads and may not know where to start and are feeling a bit intimidated. Don't worry, we're not going to leave you hanging to figure it out on your own. We've included some recipes and meal ideas to help get you started. That along with the previous list of allowed foods should help you get started on your first trip to the grocery store and to start planning meals.

Here are some favorite keto meals that should please the whole family, whether following a keto diet or a standard diet.

Breakfast Ideas

Sausage and Pepper Rings

2 bell peppers (any color)

8 large eggs

1 pound of breakfast sausage

4 Tablespoons of shredded parmesan

About 2 Tablespoons of Coconut Oil

Pepper and Salt to taste

Cut the tops and bottoms off of your bell peppers, rinse and remove the seeds.

Slice peppers into about 4 rings per pepper and put aside.

Using a small to medium size skillet, brown your breakfast sausage, breaking it up as you go. Once fully cooked, drain the excess grease and set it aside.

Add the coconut oil to the pan and heat on a medium-high heat.

Place your pepper rings into the pan and let then cook a little while the oil heats up.

Once you hear your oil start to sizzle, slowly crack an egg into each pepper ring giving it time to seal around the bottom of the ring.

Add your pepper and salt to your eggs and then add about 2 Tablespoons of sausage around the yolk in each pepper ring.

Cook your eggs as long as you like then remove them from your pan and add ½ Tablespoon of parmesan cheese to each pepper ring.

Each serving is 2 pepper rings and is about 5 grams of Net Carbs per Serving.

Roll ups

10 Large Eggs

1-1/2 cups of shredded cheddar (1/3 cup each)

5 slices of cooked bacon

5 cooked breakfast sausage patties (no sugar added)

Pepper and Salt to taste

Nonstick cooking spray

Spray your pan with nonstick cooking spray.

Pre-heat your nonstick pan over a medium-high heat.

Once your pan is hot turn it down to a medium-low heat.

Put 2 of your eggs into a bowl and whisk them together.

Add the eggs to your pan and add Pepper and Salt to your liking.

Cover your pan with a lid and allow your eggs to cook for a few minutes.

Once your eggs are almost cooked through, sprinkle about 1/3 of a cup of cheese on your eggs.

Place one strip of bacon across the middle of your eggs and then break your sausage patty in half and put it on top of the bacon.

Now, carefully roll the eggs over your fillings so that it is wrapped up like a burrito. You may have to use your spatula to hold the first side in place for a couple of seconds before it will stay to be able to fold the other side over.

Flip it over in the pan so it is folded side down and allow it to cook for a couple of seconds, this will help to keep it wrapped in place after you take it out of the pan.

Each serving is 1 Roll Up and totals out to about 2.26 Net Carbs Each.

Pancakes with Berries and Whipped Cream

4 Eggs

7 Ounces of cottage cheese

1 Tablespoon of ground psyllium husk powder

2 Ounces of butter

Topping

2 Ounces of either fresh raspberries, blueberries or strawberries

1 cup of heavy whipping cream

Add the eggs, cottage cheese, and the psyllium husk powder, to a bowl and mix together until well blended.

Once mixed, set the bowl aside for about 5-20 minutes to allow the batter to thicken.

In a nonstick skillet, melt the butter over a medium-low heat.

Pour ¼ of the batter into the pan and cook for about 3-4 minutes on each side.

Repeat for the remaining batter, making 4 pancakes.

Using another bowl, whip the heavy whipping cream until soft peaks form.

Serve the pancakes with the whipped cream and berries on top.

Serving size is 1 pancake. Each serving is 4 grams of carbs.

Breakfast Biscuit

4 ounces of pork sausage

½ cup of chopped onion

½ cup of green bell pepper chopped

¾ cup of almond flour

½ teaspoon of salt

½ teaspoon of pepper

1 teaspoon of baking powder

3 eggs

1 cup of shredded cheddar cheese

Preheat your oven to 375 degrees F.

While the oven is heating, saute the sausage, onion and pepper in a frying pan until the sausage has browned and the vegetables have softened.

Set the pan aside and let cool.

In a mixing bowl, add flour, salt, pepper and baking powder. Mix well

In a separate bowl, beat the eggs then add ½ cup of the shredded cheddar cheese and stir.

Add the egg mixture to you flour mixture and blend well.

Once the contents of the 2 bowls are mixed, add the cooled sausage, onion and pepper mixture and combine well.

Line a large cookie sheet with parchment paper.

Place large, heaping spoonfuls of the mixture about 2 inches apart on the cookie sheet.

Gently press down on each one with the back of your spoon to flatten them out just a little bit.

Sprinkle the biscuits with the remaining cheese and bake in the over for about 8-10 minutes.

Recipe makes about 12 servings. 2.9 Net carbs per serving.

Breakfast biscuits can be stored in the freezer and microwaved for about 30-60 seconds each.

Lunch Ideas

Lunches can be tough for any diet. Often lunches need to be food that travels well as it will be taken to school or to work. Some are lucky enough to have enough time and restaurants nearby where they can by a lunch that will be safe for them on this way of eating, but that can quickly become expensive and you can never be quite sure what your food is being cooked in or with, unless you do it yourself. Leftovers can make a great lunch and keep you from wasting food. Below are some quick lunch ideas you may like to try.

Stuffed Bacon Wrapped Burger

2 Tablespoons of Ghee or lard

1 sliced medium white onion

2-1/2 cups of sliced bell pepper (any color)

2 cups of white mushrooms sliced

2-1/4 pounds of ground beef

Pepper and salt to taste

10 slices of bacon (thin cut)

1-1/4 cups of shredded cheddar

5 teaspoons of sriracha

5 teaspoons of Dijon mustard

Grease your skillet with either ghee or lard.

Add the onions and cook over medium heat until lightly brown

Add your bell peppers to the onions and cook for an additional 5 minutes.

Add sliced mushrooms to your skillet and cook for 3-5 minutes.

Remove your pan from the heat.

Divide the ground beef into 5 equal parts.

Flatten each part out using your hands then take a glass and place it in the middle of the burger.

Fold the meat up around the glass making a cup or bowl out of the meat.

With the glass still in the meat, wrap 2 slices of bacon around the "meat cup".

Carefully remove the glass by twisting and pulling up.

Fill each meat cup with the cooked veggies and top with a teaspoon each of the sriracha and Dijon and a ¼ cup of shredded cheese.

Bake the cups in the oven at 300 degrees F for 45-60 minutes or until the meat has reached an internal temperature of 165 degrees.

Take them out of the oven and let them rest for 5 minutes.

Enjoys with a side of greens.

5.2 Net carbs per serving.

Turkey Taco Wrap

1 Tablespoon of Olive Oil

¾ cup of chopped yellow onion

1 pound of lean ground turkey

2 garlic cloves

Pepper and salt to taste

1 Tablespoon of chili powder

1 teaspoon of cumin

½ teaspoon of paprika

½ cup of tomato sauce (no sugar added)

½ cup of chicken broth

Romain lettuce leaves (Iceburg lettuce could also work)

Heat the olive oil in your skillet over a medium-high heat.

Add the onion and saute it for about 2 minutes.

Add the ground turkey and garlic to your pan and pepper and salt to taste.

While cooking, stir the meat mixture occasionally and break it up.

Once the meat is fully cooked, (about 5 minutes) add in your seasonings, tomato sauce and chicken broth.

Reduce heat and let simmer for about 5 minutes, occasionally stirring until the sauce has reduced.

Serve the meat mixture in the lettuce leaves.

If taking this meal to school or work, I would try to pack the lettuce separate from the meat to try to keep it crisp until lunch time.

You may also like to add toppings for your taco wrap. Shredded Mexican cheese, diced roma tomatoes, diced avocado, chopped cilantro and sour cream make great additions. Just remember to factor them in to your carb count.

Serving size is 1 taco wrap. 5 Net Carbs per Serving.

Dinner Ideas

Ranch Porkchops

6 Boneless Porkchops (thick cut)

8 ounces of full fat cream cheese (softened and cut into cubes)

8 Tablespoons of salted butter

½ cup of heavy cream

½ cup of chicken broth

3 Tablespoons of ranch seasoning (not dressing)

Pink Himalayan Sea salt to taste

Ground black pepper to taste

Season both sides of your porkchops using the sea salt and black pepper.

Heat 4 Tablespoons of butter over a medium-high heated skillet until it is melted.

Sear your porkchops for about 4-5minutes on each side until they are a golden brown color.

Reduce your heat to medium and continue to cook the porkchops until they reach an internal temperature of about 135 degrees F.

Remove the porkchops from the pan and set them aside.

Pour the chicken broth into the pan to deglaze it. Using a spatula, scrape the pan to get all of the browned pieces into the broth.

Add the cream cheese, remaining butter, and heavy cream to the pan and stir continuously until it is smooth. (Cream cheese must be softened and cut into small cubes for this to work well.)

Add the ranch seasoning and stir until it is completely combined in the sauce.

Reduce your heat to low and add your porkchops back into the pan.

Cover the pan and simmer for 10 minutes or until the porkchops reach 145 degrees.

Serve with a side of zoodles, salad or riced cauliflower.

Serving size is 1 porkchop. 0grams of Net carbs per serving. (not including a side)

Easy Pizza Casserole

2- 10 ounce packages of frozen riced cauliflower

1-1/2 cup of shredded mozzarella cheese

1 teaspoon of Italian seasoning

15 slices of pepperoni quartered, plus extra slices for the top of your casserole

Preheat the oven to 350 degrees F.

Prepare the frozen cauliflower according to the directions on the packages.

Mix the riced cauliflower with 1 cup of the mozzarella cheese, the Italian seasoning, and the 15 quartered pepperoni slices.

Pour your mixture into a baking pan.

Sprinkle the remaining mozzarella cheese on top of you casserole and finish it off with some more pepperoni slices.

Bake 20-25 minutes.

Serve with a side salad.

Serving size is ¼ of casserole. 2 grams of Net carbs per serving.

Ranch Chicken Bites

2 pounds of boneless, skinless chicken breast or thighs.

2 Tablespoons of dry ranch seasoning

2 Tablespoons of olive oil

Cut the chicken into 1" to 2" chunks.

Put them in a bowl with 1 Tablespoon of olive oil and the ranch seasoning.

Stir until the chicken is well coated.

Cover the bowl with plastic wrap and place it in the fridge for about 15 minutes to allow the flavors to combine.

Heat the remaining 1 Tablespoon of oil in a skillet over high heat.

Add the chicken and spread into an even flat layer in the pan.

Allow the chicken to cook for about 4 to 5 minutes without moving it.

Then flip the pieces over and cook and additional 3 to 5 minutes until the chicken is cooked through.

Serve the chicken hot with your favorite side dish such as a salad or vegetable. This chicken would be great over a salad once allowed to cool.

Each serving is about ½ pound. Each serving contains 1 gram of Net carbs.

Crack Chicken Casserole

2 cups of cooked chicken, chopped

½ pound of cooked bacon, chopped

4 large eggs

1 cup of shredded cheddar cheese

½ cup of heavy cream

½ cup of full fat ranch dressing

Nonstick cooking spray

Preheat your oven to 350 degrees F.

Lightly spray and 8" by 8" pan with nonstick cooking spray.

Spread the cooked chicken and bacon out across the bottom of the pan.

Top the chicken and bacon with the shredded cheese.

In a medium sized bowl, whisk together the eggs, ranch dressing and heavy cream.

Pour on top of the chicken mixture.

Bake uncovered for 30 to 35 minutes.

Recipe makes 6 servings. Each serving contains about 1.5 Net carbs.

Snack Ideas

Parmesan Crisps

¾ cup of shredded parmesan cheese

¾ cup of shredded cheddar cheese

1 tsp of Italian Seasoning (optional)

Preheat your oven to 400 degrees F.

Line a large cookie sheet with parchment paper.

While the oven is still preheating, stir your cheeses together in a small bowl.

Once cheeses are well mixed, place tablespoon sized mounds of the cheese blend onto the cookie sheet about 2 inches apart.

Sprinkle your seasoning over the cheese.

Place your cookie sheet into the oven and let it bake for about 6-8 minutes, just until the edges start to brown.

Take your cheese out of the oven and allow it time to cool in the pan before transferring onto paper towels to drain and crisp up.

Serving size is ¼ of recipe. Each serving has 1gram of Net carbs.

You can also make this recipe with just parmesan or just cheddar by just doubling the cheese of your choice. Keep and eye on them in the oven, once they start to brown they will burn quickly.

No Crust Pizza

This is a really fast an easy snack option that is completely customizable. Just have all of your ingredients ready before adding the cheese to the pan because this truly takes no time to cook!

Preheat nonstick skillet over medium heat. (nonstick is key)

Fill an area the size you would like your pizza with shredded mozzarella.

Add some parmesan cheese on top of that it you would like the added flavor.

Once the cheese starts to melt, add your toppings. Don't go too thick with them because they will not get much time to cook.

Once the edges of your cheese are brown it is ready. Either slide it out of the pan or use a spatula to get under it and remove it from the pan.

This has a great crispy "crust" and really gives you that flavor of pizza. You will have to track what you put on it to calculate your macros. More meat will mean less carbs.

Dessert Ideas

Chocolate Fat Bombs

1 cup of coconut oil

1 cup of almond butter

½ cup of unsweetened cocoa powder

4 Tablespoons of coconut flour

4 Tablespoons of raw nuts (such as almonds or cashews) chopped

Heat the coconut and the almond butter in a small pot over a medium heat and mix well, stirring frequently.

Pour the mixture into a freezer safe bowl and mix in the cocoa powder and the coconut flour.

Cover and freeze for about 1 hour or until your chocolate mixture is solid.

Once solid, remove the bowl from the freezer and scoop out about ½ teaspoon balls and roll them into the nuts to cover them.

Let them rest on a cool plate while you shape and cover the rest of the mixture.

Refrigerate the fat bombs for at least 15 minutes before serving.

Fat bombs will stay fresh in your refrigerator for up to 2 weeks in an air tight container.

Each Fat Bomb contains approximately 2 Net Carbs.

Lemon Cheesecake

Crust

1-1/4 cup of almond flour

3 Tablespoons of melted butter

1-1/2 teaspoon of Splenda or Swerve

Nonstick cooking spray

Filling

8 ounces of softened cream cheese

½ teaspoon of vanilla extract

1-1/2 cups of heavy whipping cream

.3 ounce box of sugar free lemon gelatin (or any flavor you'd prefer)

1 teaspoon of lemon zest

Preheat your oven to 350 degrees F.

Spray an 8" baking dish or a springform pan with nonstick cooking spray.

Mix the almond flour, butter and Splenda until the mixture is well combined and crumbly.

Press the mixture into the bottom of your baking dish and bake in your preheated over for about 8-10 minutes until it reaches a nice golden brown color.

Remove the pan from the oven and let it cool completely.

Using an electric mixer with a whisk attachment, mix the softened cream cheese until smooth.

Stir the vanilla extract into your cream cheese.

Add the heavy cream and whisk the mixture on high until it thickens and soft peaks have formed.

Reduce the speed on your mixer to low and add in you flavored gelatin and lemon zest. Mix until all ingredients are well combined.

Spread the creamy mixture evenly over your cooled crust using a spatula.

Cover and chill in the refrigerator for at least 2-3 hours until fully set.

Serves 6-8. Each serving contains 4.4 grams of Net Carbs.

As you can see the ketogenic diet can be very diverse and allow you to eat many different types of flavorful meals. While most meals are based around meats there are also many vegetarian options available as well although it can be slightly more difficult to reach the necessary levels of fat needed for nutritional ketosis. Because this way of eating has become so popular there are many recipes available online, just make sure to look them over carefully because as we have learned, there are many different versions of keto and you will want to make sure they fit into the version you are living.

Get creative. Play with your food. Try new combinations and new flavors. Casseroles are great for leftovers or make ahead meals when you know you won't have much time. Most can just be thrown together with left over meat like chicken, some cream cheese, heavy cream bacon and shredded cheese. Add some seasoning and you have a new meal. It really doesn't have to be complicated. Even just adding some shredded cheese and bacon or pepperoni to leftover chicken and make you feel like you're eating something different within no time at all. Once you get the hang of where your fats come from and what has carbs, you will love the simplicity of this diet.

Most diets have taught you to trim your meats before cooking them. This is not really a diet where you want to do that all of the time. Lean meats are great and offer lots of benefits and if you plan on cooking in a high fat sauce or oil, or pairing it with a side dish that is higher in fat you may want to consider trimming your meat or skinning your chicken. Otherwise, it is best to leave the skin on your chicken and not to trim your meat before cooking. You could allow the fat to render for added flavor or enjoy it as is. Let the skin of the chicken crisp up for added texture. You could even cook just the skins to have as crackling on the side to add fat to another dish or just to snack on. Depending upon where you live, it may be difficult to find meats that have not been trimmed already as although the ketogenic diet is becoming more popular, it is still more common for people to look for low fat options, an unfortunately this includes your meats. If you buy your meat from a grocery store you may not have the option, but if there is a butcher, make friends, let them know what you are looking for. They may be able to sell you cuts of meat before it is trimmed. It doesn't hurt to ask.

Chapter 6 - Desserts and Fat Bombs

What could be better than losing weight and still enjoying your favorite desserts? On a ketogenic diet you have endless options of desserts you can choose from as long as you stick with keto approved foods. (high fat, low carb) It's still not a great idea to eat cake everyday if your main goal is weight loss, but making room for it every now and then won't hurt you at all either. (sometimes it will even help you meet your fat macros)

On a ketogenic diet you have many options when it comes to food choices and the path you want to take while on this diet plan. If you enjoy sweet foods every now and then or even just on special occasions or holidays, there are options for you to help keep you on track and in ketosis. If you prefer savory foods and love to snack when relaxing to watch a movie or even just after work, there is plenty for you to eat. With a little planning you will be able to stick with the diet no matter what comes up.

But planning is the key. We all know it is those quick, sugary carbs that we reach for when we just need a quick snack to hold us over until our next meal or to just fulfill that habit of needing to eat while watching tv. If you know this is you, you have plenty of options to keep on hand when the need strikes. If the food is already made and just waiting to be eaten in the fridge, on the counter or even in the freezer, the chances of you passing by the high carb, easy and familiar food to reach for the low carb ready to eat food is much greater.

So, plan ahead, whether you take an hour or two out of your weekend, or shop with the intent to have snacks on hand that are ready to eat, (such as sugar free gelatin) just get it done. Whether you have sweet snacks or savory snacks or a little bit of both, just be prepared for when the craving hits. Often you will find the longer you follow a ketogenic lifestyle, the less you look for snacks and won't have to keep them on hand all of the time. (Unless you want to.)

And really, what other diet allows you to feed all of your sweet cravings? You will find there are countless recipes available to you that are approved for a ketogenic lifestyle. Many of your favorite desserts can be made keto friendly by just swapping out a few ingredients. Remove your all purpose flours and substitute an almond or any nut flour, switch out your sugar with a Xylitol or Stevia and you'll be off to a good start. Get creative! Experiment in the kitchen to find your favorite flour or sugar supplement. You'll soon learn what you need to make a great tasting dessert, whether just for one or the whole family. You'll find many of the recipes are even Thanksgiving worthy!

No matter what you are looking for, just about every type of dessert, from ice cream to donuts, cookies and pies can all be made low carb and they still taste amazing. You would never know they were sugar free! No matter what your skill level is in the kitchen there are desserts for you. Whether, you LOVE to bake and have no problem spending the whole day in the kitchen or prefer to just mix up a couple of ingredients for a no bake snack or fat bomb. You will even find that you can purchase all types of keto friendly desserts and chocolates online and the keto way of eating has become so popular there are now keto friendly ice cream flavors available in most grocery stores, making it even easier when that craving hits or even when you just don't want to stand out as the only one not enjoying any at the party.

Some favorite dessert options...

Creamy Chocolate Mousse

2 ounces of cream cheese (softened)

2 ounces of unsalted butter (softened)

1 Tablespoon of cocoa powder

3 ounces of heavy whipping cream

Stevia (to taste)

Combine the butter with Stevia (a little can go a long way). Continue stirring until fully blended.

Add cream cheese to your butter and sweetener and continue to blend until smooth.

Now, add your cocoa powder and stir until ingredients are completely blended.

Whip the heavy cream and slowly add it to the mixture, stirring it in as you go.

Spoon equal amounts of your mousse into 4 small glasses and refrigerate for at least 30 minutes.

Each serving contains 1.5 grams of Net carbs.

Not a fan of chocolate? Want something sweet to snack on but don't want to take the time to bake or heat up your house? Try a 3 ingredient, no bake cookie. For a softer cookie, try it at room temperature. If you crave a thicker, fudgy texture, you can eat these straight out of the fridge.

No Bake Coconut Cookies

You'll need

3 cups of unsweetened, shredded coconut flakes

1 cup of melted coconut oil

½ cup monk fruit sweetened maple syrup

Line a large baking pan or platter with parchment paper and set it aside.

Add all ingredients to a large bowl and mix until well combined.

Using slightly wet hands, form small balls out of the mixture and place them about 2 inches apart on your parchment lined platter.

Now using a fork, press down on top of each cookie to flatten it out on your platter.

Refrigerate cookies until firm.

These cookies will keep for 7 days in air tight container at room temperature or can be refrigerated for up to a month.

Serving size is 1 cookie. Each cookie is 0 grams of Net carbs.

Do you miss candy bars? Need a lower carb alternative for when that craving hits?

Try this no bake option.

Caramel Almond Chocolate Bars

<u>For the chocolate layer you'll need:</u>

1-1/2 cups of dark chocolate chips

1 Tablespoon of butter

2 Tablespoons of heavy cream at room temperature

<u>To make the caramel you will need:</u>

4 Tablespoons of butter

¼ cup of xylitol

½ cup of heavy cream

Chopped roasted peanuts for topping

Salt to taste

<u>For the almond layer you'll need:</u>

1 cup of almond flour

¼ cup of sugar free almond butter

1 Tablespoon of monk fruit or your favorite keto sweetener

Starting with the chocolate layer, melt the butter and dark chocolate using either a double boiler or the microwave.

Stir in the heavy cream.

Pour it into a small baking dish lined with wax paper or parchment.

Next, in a medium bowl stir together all the ingredients in the almond layer.

It should be able to hold itself together. If not, add a small amount more of almond butter to help make it stickier.

Add it into the chocolate and lightly press it down into an even layer.

Place the dish into t he freezer to allow it to harden.

Next, to make the caramel you will need to add the butter to a small sauce pan and heat over a medium/low heat and bring it to a simmer.

Be sure to stir the butter often and allow it to become browned.

Add in the sweetener, salt and heavy cream and stir until fully combined.

Simmer over a very low heat for about 15 minutes but do not stir.

Once done, allow your caramel to cool then remove your layers from the freezer.

Pour the caramel over your layers of chocolate and almond butter then sprinkle with chopped peanuts.

Cut your dessert into 6 bars.

Serving size is 1 bar. Each serving contains 6grams of Net carbs.

Keto Ice Cream

2 cups of canned full fat coconut milk

1/3 cup of xylitol or your favorite keto friendly sweetener

1-1/2 teaspoon of vanilla extract

1/8 teaspoon of salt

In a large bowl stir together the milk, salt, vanilla extract and sweetener.

If you have an ice cream machine you can churn the mixture.

If you do not have an ice cream maker, simply pour the mixture into ice cream trays.

Put the trays in the freezer and allow to freeze.

Blend the cubes in a blender or allow them to thaw some to be able to mix in a food processor.

You can then eat it as is or put back int the freezer if you prefer a firmer texture.

You can experiment with different flavors by adding additional ingredients such as frozen strawberries, cocoa powder, or even coffee frozen into ice cubes.

This recipe makes about 4-5 servings. Each serving has about 1 Net carb

You can make some even easier desserts using the individual cups of sugar free gelatin.

Choose any flavor you like and top it with 2 Tablespoons of Rediwhip for a dessert with just 1 gram of carbs per serving.

You can also change it up a bit by whipping them together for a more mousse-like dessert. Or mixing them up and freezing them in popsicle molds for a nice summer treat.

Let's not forget about fat bombs! Fat bombs are a delicious keto treat that can be a very important part of your diet. They will help you reach your macro goals using healthy fats while keeping your carbs low. These bite size snacks can be made ahead of time so they can always available to you when you are hungry or are craving something sweet. Keeping fat bombs on hand will keep you from being tempted by high carb, sugary sweets. What exactly is a fat bomb? Fat bombs are at least 80% fat, many are more than 90% fat and are made with a high fat base such as coconut oil or cream cheese, keto approved sweeteners and just a small amount of protein. Especially when you are still new to a keto diet it can be difficult to attain the high fat percentages needed to be able to reach and maintain a healthy state of ketosis. You may often find that you are just too full to eat another meal but still are falling short on your fat macros. Because they are a small snack with a high concentration of fat they will help you reach your goals and provide you with the energy needed to finish your day strong.

Fat bombs start with a chosen fat such as butter, cream cheese, or coconut oil and then add in your favorite flavors such as almond butter, cocoa powder or lemon and vanilla with a small amount of zero calorie sweetener like erythritol or sucralose. Mix your ingredients together, mold and refrigerate them. You can made them into balls or rolls, or even use candy molds. Ice cube trays make great molds for bite sized fat bombs as well as mini cupcake pans. Most fat bomb recipes you find are sweet but you can even make a more savory treat by experimenting with animal fats like lard or tallow and adding bacon bits, chopped meats such as steak or salami and herbs and spices. The only limit is your imagination and since they take no time at all to mix up you can try lots of different combinations until you find your favorites.

Do you have a busy day ahead of you? Don't know how you will find the time to fit lunch in? You can even get creative and make a meal replacement fat bomb, such as a pizza fat bomb using cream cheese and some of your favorite pizza toppings chopped and mixed in. Or a breakfast replacement bomb using cream cheese and mixing in hard boiled eggs and bacon. You could pack up a couple of these options to take with you to eat on the go.

Garlic Cheddar Fat Bomb

6 ounces of slightly softened cream cheese

6 ounces of shredded cheddar

¾ teaspoon of garlic powder

1 Tablespoon of minced parsley

½ teaspoon of dried dill

5 Tablespoons of chopped pecans

In a medium sized bowl, mix together the cheddar, cream cheese, dried dill and garlic powder. Stir until well combined.

Place plastic wrap on top of your cheese mixture and allow to cool in freezer for about 8 minutes.

Remove the bowl from the freezer and separate the mixture evenly into 14 balls.

Combine the parsley and chopped pecans in a small shallow bowl and roll each ball into the mixture to cover.

These fat bombs work great as a snack or even a side to your meal. You can store them in the fridge for up to a week in an airtight container.

Makes 14 servings. Each serving contains 0 grams of Net carbs.

Mediterranean Fat Bombs

½ cup of cream cheese

¼ cup of softened butter or ghee

2-3 Tablespoons of freshly chopped herbs such as basil, thyme and oregano or use your favorites!

4 pieces of drained sun dried tomatoes

4 pitted olives

2 cloves of crushed garlic

Ground black pepper to taste

Pink Himalayan sea salt to taste

5 Tablespoons of parmesan cheese

Cut your butter into small pieces and put it in a bowl with the cream cheese. Allow it to sit out at room temperature for about 30 minutes to soften so that it will be easier to work with.

Once softened, mix the butter and cream cheese together with the sun dried tomatoes and olives until well combined.

Add your herbs, crushed garlic, salt and pepper and continue mixing.

Once ingredients are mixed, place the bowl in the fridge for about 20 to 30 minutes to allow it to solidify.

Add your parmesan cheese to a plate or shallow bowl.

Remove your cheese mixture from the fridge and roll it into 5 balls.

Roll each ball into the parmesan cheese to coat it.

Your fat bombs are now ready to enjoy, or they can be stored int the fridge for up to one week in an airtight container.

Recipe makes 5 servings. Each serving contains 1.7 grams of Net carbs.

For something a little sweeter you could also try…

Chocolate Peanut Butter Fat Bombs

4 Tablespoons of butter

4 Tablespoons of peanut butter

4 Tablespoons of refined coconut oil

2 Tablespoons of unsweetened cocoa powder

Sweeten to taste using Stevia or your favorite keto sweetener

Melt your butter in a microwave safe bowl.

Add peanut butter, cocoa powder and coconut oil and blend well using a mixer or immersion blender.

Add sweetener to taste.

Pour into candy molds or ice cube trays and freeze for 20 minutes.

Fat bombs should be stored in the freezer in airtight container.

Makes 24 servings. Each serving contains 1 Net carb.

Salted Caramel and Peanut Butter Fat Bombs

8 Tablespoons of unsalted butter

1 cup of natural chunky peanut butter

¼ cup of sugar free Salted Caramel Syrup

1 cup of coconut oil

In a sauce pan, melt all ingredients over a medium heat stirring often.

Once all ingredients have melted and are well combined, pour them into silicone molds or an ice cube tray and freeze.

Once fat bombs have set, remove from their molds and store them in an airtight container in the freezer.

Recipe makes 18 servings. Each serving contains 1.9 grams of Net carbs.

Not a fan of peanut butter? Try these.

Strawberry Cheesecake Fat Bombs

¾ cups of cream cheese

¼ cup of butter

½ cup of fresh or frozen strawberries

1 teaspoon of vanilla extract

2 Tablespoons of heavy cream

8 drops of alcohol free stevia

Cut both the cream cheese and the butter into cubes, place in a bowl and allow it to sit at room temperature for about an hour until softened.

Mash the strawberries with a fork or blender if frozen and set aside.

Using and electric mixer, combine the cream cheese, butter, vanilla, heavy cream and stevia until well combined.

Add the strawberries to your mix and stir in by hand.

Spoon the mix into candy molds or ice cube trays and freeze for 2 to 3 hours until solid.

Remove from molds and store in airtight container in the freezer.

Recipe makes 12 servings. 1 gram of Net carbs per serving.

It's hard to believe that eating this much fat will help you lose weight, but as long as you stay away from the high carbs your body will stay in ketosis and keep you from storing that fat. It's only when you are mixing these high fat foods with a high carb diet that your body will burn off the carbs for energy and just continue to store the fat making you gain weight. Keto is an all or nothing diet. You cannot just add in the high fat foods (no matter how delicious) and keep to your hi carb ways and see results. Your body will never reach a state of ketosis and you will just find yourself gaining more weight. It doesn't have to be difficult, you don't need to make fancy, multi-step meals everyday. You just have to decide to stick with it, and to help you on your journey to weight loss and a new way of eating we have included a 30 day meal plan to keep you from having to figure out what to eat everyday.

Chapter 7 - 30 Day Meal Plan

Changing over to a ketogenic diet from a more conventional way of eating can seem overwhelming at first, but it doesn't have to be. Start out with a plan to reduce carbs and increase fats. While for most capping their carbohydrate intake at 50 grams will be enough for them to reach ketosis, others will have to reduce even further, sometimes to as low as 20 grams of net carbs to achieve a nutritional state of ketosis. You won't know until you try.

For most households you will need to go out and purchase foods and ingredients you may have never eaten before. Take some time to create a meal plan, or use the one provided. Make a shopping list and give yourself some extra time to shop on your first couple of trips. Not only are you going to be looking for new ingredients that you may have never seen before, but you will also need some time to check labels once you do find something that you THINK you want to buy. While trying new foods and recipes helps add a variety to your diet as well as additional nutrients you may not be getting in the typical foods you are comfortable eating, it is not absolutely necessary to go out and purchase new types of flour or sweeteners. But that doesn't mean you can use your traditional high carb ingredients either. It just means that rather than using a keto friendly almond flour to make a pizza crust or dessert, you now, skip that dessert recipe or try a crustless pizza or even a chicken based pizza crust. Some of these recipes and foods may take you out of your comfort zone, but it is because of that food that made you so comfortable that you are now looking for a new way of eating to be able to lose weight and feel better. Try going into this diet with an open mind. Of course you will not like every new food you try, but you might be surprised by the ones you do like. Without giving them a chance, you'll never know. So, venture out, even if you only try one new food per week and stick to basic meat with added fat and vegetables the rest of the time, you will find there is much more out there than what you have been eating, and I bet you'll find some new favorite recipes to add into your family's rotation.

So, do you feel well prepared to start your journey to this new way of life? Have all of your questions been answered? It's time to get started then!

Included in the previous chapters are some recipes that you can swap in for any meal, but to make it easy when starting out, this meal plan will include just the basics of the meal. You can add your own seasonings and cook the meat as you like whether it be on the grill, baked or in the frying pan. If you are already using a leaner cut of meat it would be best to cook it in a frying pan with added fat to help you attain your macros. There is no calorie guide, listen to your body and stop eating when you are full. Track your macros daily and adjust accordingly. Remember fat is the focus and 5% carbs is your max. A snack has been included in the meal plan each day. You may not want a snack every day and especially as you become more fat adapted you will not need one. When you want one, have one. Otherwise, skip it. And fat bombs can be used just about any day if you find you are a little short on your fats for the day. They are great to always keep on hand, ready to eat, whether with a meal or after dinner as a dessert. Enjoy your food and your new body!

Day 1

For Breakfast:

Scrambled eggs (no milk) cooked in butter with a side of bacon.

For Lunch:

Turkey Taco Wrap (recipe included in chapter 5)

For Dinner:

Fatty steak and salad

As a Snack:

Macadamia Nuts

<u>Day 2</u>

For Breakfast:

Feta cheese and spinach omelet cooked in butter

For Lunch:

Cheeseburger lettuce wrap

For Dinner:

Grilled shrimp with a sauce of melted butter and lemon and a side of asparagus

As a Snack:

Parmesan Crisps (recipe included in chapter 5)

<u>Day 3</u>

For Breakfast:

Sausage Egg Muffins

For Lunch:

Deli Meat Roll Ups with bell pepper strips (make sure to use quality deli meats with little to no fillers)

For Dinner:

Ranch Porkchops with a side of zoodles (recipe included in chapter 5)

As a Snack:

Fat bomb

Day 4

For Breakfast:

Pancakes with cream and berries (recipe included in chapter 5)

For Lunch:

Grilled chicken salad with olive oil dressing

For Dinner:

Saute kielbasa and cabbage in butter with diced onion, garlic and seasonings

As a Snack:

Pork rinds dipped in sour cream

Day 5

For Breakfast:

Eggs fried in butter with a side of sausage

For Lunch:

Chicken wings baked in butter and seasoning with side salad

For Dinner:

Pizza Casserole (recipe included in chapter 5)

As a Snack:

Chocolate Mousse

<u>Day 6</u>

For Breakfast:

Sausage and Pepper Rings (recipe included in chapter 5)

For Lunch:

Stuffed Bacon Wrapped Burger (recipe included in chapter 5)

For Dinner:

Chicken thighs with a side of zucchini

As a Snack:

No crust pepperoni pizza (recipe included in chapter 5)

<u>Day 7</u>

For Breakfast:

Pancakes and bacon (recipe included in chapter 5)

For Lunch:

Grilled chicken lettuce wrap and zucchini chips

For Dinner:

Meatloaf with a side of broccoli (use crushed pork rinds in place of bread crumbs)

As a Snack:

Caramel Almond Bar (recipe included in chapter 6)

You made it through your first week! You may have started to feel the beginnings of the keto flu. Remember, drink plenty of water and get some rest. You'll be feeling better soon.

<u>Day 8</u>

For Breakfast:

Breakfast Roll Up (recipe included in chapter 5)

For Lunch:

Ground Turkey Taco Salad (recipe included in chapter 5)

For Dinner:

Roast sliced sausages with veggies in sheet pan with olive oil.

As a Snack:

Cheese slices

Day 9

For Breakfast:

Sausage and bacon omelet cooked in butter

For Lunch:

Chicken fajita wrapped in lettuce

For Dinner:

Pot Roast and riced cauliflower

As a Snack:

Fat Bomb

Day 10

For Breakfast:

Pancakes with cream and berries (recipe included in chapter 5)

For Lunch:

Cheeseburger lettuce wrap

For Dinner:

Baked chicken thighs topped with cheese and bacon with green beans

As a Snack:

No bake Coconut Cookie (recipe included in chapter 6)

<u>Day 11</u>

For Breakfast:

Scrambled eggs cooked in butter with side of bacon

For Lunch:

Grilled chicken salad

For Dinner:

"Nachos" Top pork rinds with seasoned ground beef or turkey, cheese and sour cream

As a Snack:

Chocolate Mousse (recipe included in chapter 6)

<u>Day 12</u>

For Breakfast:

Sausage Pancake Roll Up (recipe included in chapter 5)

For Lunch:

Chicken wings with zucchini chips

For Dinner:

Steak and asparagus topped with garlic butter

As a Snack:

Parmesan crisps

<u>Day 13</u>

For Breakfast:

Breakfast bowl with egg, sausage and bacon

For Lunch:

Turkey Taco Wrap (recipe included in chapter 5)

For Dinner:

Steak and veggie skewer with riced cauliflower

As a Snack:

Fat bomb

<u>Day 14</u>

For Breakfast:

Celery dipped in almond butter

For Lunch:

Bacon wrapped cheeseburger

For Dinner:

Seasoned chicken thighs with garlic butter zoodles

As a Snack:

Salami

You made it through week 2! Hopefully, you are starting to feel better and gaining energy. Some may just be starting to feel the flu now. Don't give up yet. Remember to stay hydrated and if you are not hungry, don't eat. You don't need to have the snacks every day!

<u>Day 15</u>

For Breakfast:

Strawberries and cream pancakes (recipe included in chapter 5)

For Lunch:

Deli meat and cheese roll up (remember to choose a quality deli meat with little to no fillers)

For Dinner:

Ranch Porkchops with cauliflower and broccoli (recipe included in chapter 5)

As a Snack:

Fat Bomb

Day 16

For Breakfast:

Sausage and Pepper Rings (recipe included in chapter 5)

For Lunch:

Grilled Chicken Salad with Olive Oil dressing

For Dinner:

Steak with asparagus and garlic butter sauce

As a Snack:

Macadamia Nuts

For Breakfast:

Sausage, egg and cheese breakfast bowl

For Lunch:

Deli meat Roll Ups with zucchini chips (choose a quality deli meat with little to no fillers)

For Dinner:

Pizza Casserole (recipe included in chapter 5)

As a Snack:

No bake coconut cookie (recipe included in chapter 6)

Day 18

For Breakfast:

Breakfast Biscuit (recipe included in chapter 5)

For Lunch:

Turkey Taco Salad (recipe included in chapter 5)

For Dinner:

Pot Roast with broccoli

As a Snack:

Chocolate mousse (recipe included in chapter 6)

Day 19

For Breakfast:

Pancakes with sausage (recipe included in chapter 5)

For Lunch:

Grilled chicken fajita lettuce wrap

For Dinner:

Porkchops and salad

As a Snack:

Sugar free gelatin with whipped cream

Day 20

For Breakfast:

Sausage, Bacon and cheese omelet

For Lunch:

Stuffed bacon wrapped burger with bell pepper strips (recipe included in chapter 5)

For Dinner:

Sauteed shrimp in buttered zoodles

As a Snack:

Baked pepperoni chips

<u>Day 21</u>

For Breakfast:

Pancakes and sausage (recipe included in chapter 5)

For Lunch:

Chicken veggie wrap

For Dinner:

Pizza Casserole (recipe included in chapter 5)

As a Snack:

Fat Bomb

It takes 21 days to create a habit and you have just completed 3 weeks on a ketogenic diet! Have you found any new foods that you LOVE yet? You should be feeling a bit more energized now as you are becoming fat adapted. Your flu should be just about gone by now and you may even be finding that you are not as hungry as often or you forgot to eat lunch. You should have seen some weight loss by now too, maybe even need to go out to buy new pants.

Day 22

For Breakfast:

Breakfast biscuit (recipe included in chapter 5)

For Lunch:

Turkey Taco Wrap (recipe included in chapter 5)

For Dinner:

Sausage and veggies roasted in olive oil

As a Snack:

Pork rinds dipped in sour cream

Day 23

For Breakfast:

Scrambled eggs cooked in butter with side of sausage

For Lunch:

Cheeseburger wrapped in lettuce with parmesan crisps

For Dinner:

Pork roast with sauteed vegetables

As a Snack:

Fat Bomb

Day 24

For Breakfast:

Breakfast Roll Ups (recipe included in chapter 5)

For Lunch:

Roasted chicken and vegetables

For Dinner:

Beef and broccoli stir fry with cauliflower rice

As a Snack:

Chocolate mousse (recipe included in chapter 6)

<u>Day 25</u>

For Breakfast:

Pancakes with cream and berries (recipe included in chapter 5)

For Lunch:

Chicken fajita wrap

For Dinner:

Pizza Casserole (recipe included in chapter 5)

As a Snack:

Fat Bomb

<u>Day 26</u>

For Breakfast:

Sausage and Pepper Rings (recipe included in chapter 5)

For Lunch:

Grilled chicken salad with olive oil dressing

For Dinner:

Meatloaf and mashed cauliflower or green beans (substitute crushed pork rinds for the bread crumbs)

As a Snack:

Sugar free gelatin with whipped cream

<u>Day 27</u>

For Breakfast:

Breakfast Roll Ups (recipe included in chapter 5)

For Lunch:

Cheeseburger wrapped in lettuce with zucchini chips

For Dinner:

Chicken thigh with roasted vegetables

As a Snack:

Fat bomb

<u>Day 28</u>

For Breakfast:

Sausage, egg and cheese breakfast bowl

For Lunch:

Chicken wings with a side of parmesan crisps

For Dinner:

Steak and Asparagus

As a Snack:

Almonds

Day 29

For Breakfast:

Breakfast Biscuit (recipe included in chapter 5)

For Lunch:

Turkey Taco Wrap (recipe included in chapter 5)

For Dinner:

Shrimp in garlic butter zoodles

As a Snack:

Fat bomb

Day 30

For Breakfast:

Pancakes with cream and berries (recipe included in chapter 5)

For Lunch:

Cheeseburger lettuce wrap

For Dinner:

Baked chicken topped with cheese and bacon with a side of mashed cauliflower

As a Snack:

No bake coconut cookie (recipe included in chapter 5)

You did it! You have just completed 30 days on a ketogenic diet. You should be in a state of ketosis and burning fat for energy. If you are not sure you can check by using some ketone test strips available at your local pharmacy. They are usually low priced but not really necessary if you have already noticed any of the symptoms of ketosis. Now that you have become fat adapted it would be a good time to start the 16/8 method of intermittent fasting to help increase your weight loss even more. Just figure out the best time of day for your meal period and get started. It really is as easy as that.

Keto milkshakes are a great option to substitute in on a busy day. You could mix equal amounts of heavy cream and water with some crushed ice and cocoa powder plus a little sweetener for something basic. Or you can add in a little nut butter or seeds for a different taste and texture. Some almond milk with heavy cream and a few strawberries would be great too. It doesn't have to be complicated. You can even mix it up the night before if you don't have time in the morning. I would try to blend in the ice just before drinking though if possible if you like it to be a bit thicker. They tend to get a bit thin overnight.

Also, you will find that unflavored pork rinds (flavored usually contain some form of sugar) are very versatile. You can snack on them right out of the bag but they are high in protein so watch your serving sizes. But they can also be crushed to replace bread crumbs in many recipes. They work in meatloaf and meatballs, but you can also use them as a coating on chicken or pork shops before baking or pan frying. Mixing them with fresh parmesan cheese and seasonings can add new flavors and textures you your everyday foods.

Chapter 8 - Tips and Tricks to Help You Stay on Track

Keto doesn't have to be difficult and can easily fit into any lifestyle. It is very easy to meal plan and make a couple of dishes or fat bombs ahead of time and pack them up to take to work to help keep you from feeling tempted when hungry. No time to pack a lunch? Most fast food restaurants have keto friendly foods when in a bind. Plain bunless burger patties are usually the safest option. Most fast food restaurants have a plan to package patties only with no bun and many will give you a discount on it too, although you might have to ask. Be careful with the cheese and bacon at some of these restaurants. Most are processed cheeses and the bacon may be high in sugar as well as nitrates and nitrites. When going out to dinner with friends it's usually easiest to start with the gluten free menu and go from there. Again, ketogenic diets have become very popular so most restaurants can accommodate a low carb, no sugar meal. Just ask for whichever meat you would like and get it without the sauce, add vegetables as your side and you will have a complete meal that just about any restaurant can handle.

There are many meal trackers and macro counters available online and in app stores. Find one that works well for you and has a convenient method to add your food. It's always easier to use an app that allows you to just scan the barcode for the product you want to add. Remember though, that many trackers allow users to upload nutrition information and trackers can vary greatly. If the numbers don't seem correct, check another source or verify the nutrition label whenever possible. You don't want to be pushed out of ketosis due to someone else's error in logging nutrition facts.

We've already established that you can get into a state of ketosis fairly quickly by fasting. (especially if you have already been in ketosis and your body has become used to burning fat for energy) If you make a mistake and knock yourself out of ketosis don't beat yourself up too much. Just get yourself back on track right away. The easiest way would be to fast. Fasting for at least 24 hours (longer if you can) then eating a large fatty steak will help get your body burning fat again. During your fasting period your body should run through whatever carbs you ingested that caused you to fall out of ketosis and if fasting long enough your body will have to start working on your fat stores again to keep it energized. Feeding it a fatty steak that doesn't have any carbs continues to fuel your body but doesn't add to any of the glucose that may be leftover. You should feel the difference again soon. I just wouldn't recommend doing it often so as to not have to go through an adaptation period again. Also, if you are new to fasting, try to take it easy during your fast. Don't over exert yourself or try a new workout. Your body will be working hard as it is, no need to add stress.

Holidays, parties, and special events! You don't have to miss out on the fun of these social events. Most parties and holidays revolve around food and drinks, while you may have to be more selective now, there is still plenty you can join in on. Plan on enjoying the meats at any of your gatherings, just steer clear of the sauces and gravies as most will be made with sugars and flour. Most side dishes during the holidays are very carb heavy so look for salads and veggie trays. Speak to the host ahead of time if you are comfortable telling people about your way of eating. Now that it is more popular many are familiar with some sort of low carb way of eating. Offer to bring a dish to share so that you know there will always be at least one thing you can eat at the party. If really unsure, or uncomfortable asking to bring food, eat before you go that way if you don't end up eating much (or anything) at the gathering you won't be too hungry to enjoy the night out. Think about hosting the holidays yourself. This will allow you to control all of the food and mix in keto versions of your traditional meals and maybe even introduce new foods or lower carb options to your friends and family.

Wondering if you can still drink alcohol while on the keto diet? Well, the answer is yes. But you will have to watch which drinks you choose, and it may affect your weight loss results. Raising your blood alcohol level can cause your body to crave carb heavy foods. When you're not thinking clearly, it may not be as easy for you to make the best decisions. Also, when your body doesn't have any carbs to soak up the alcohol, it's especially easy to get drunk, so be sure you are in a safe place and don't have to drive anywhere. Your liver treats alcohol as a toxin so it will take you out of ketosis while it puts all of its energy into filtering it out of your blood. If you don't drink often you will have time to get back into ketosis but remember, it can take days to weeks for that to happen depending on what you choose to drink. Dry red or white wines usually total about 2 grams of carbs per glass. Beer is usually high in carbs and is made with grains and yeast so not the best option. Hard alcohol has zero carbs if you stick to the unflavored such as whiskey, tequila, rum and vodka. A cocktail out of sugar free lemonade and some vodka may help keep you from feeling left out on the fun and keep you from adding carbs. Just take it slow until you know how your body will react. Maybe plan to exercise in the morning to help burn off any lingering carbs.

Use plenty of coconut oil when just starting out on your diet. Coconut oil will help to provide you with the healthy fat you need as well as containing MCTs. MCTs are taken directly to your liver to immediately be used for energy or converted to be stored as ketones. It will help increase your ketone levels and allow you to burn more fat, but be careful with how much you use as it can cause digestive discomfort such as stomach cramping and diarrhea.

Once you have become fat adapted work in some time for exercise. If you can add your work out in while still in a fasted state research has shown that it can increase your ketone levels by up to 300%.

It cannot be stressed enough, getting enough sleep and allowing your body time to recover especially during the adaptation phase is extremely important. Let it rest so that it will have the energy needed to burn fat and convert to ketones.

Many fat bombs and keto desserts as well as keto meals will keep well in the fridge or freezer. If you are the only one in your household on this way of eating you can still make full batches of your favorite meals and just split them up into individual sized meals before putting them in the fridge or freezer, allowing you to just take out the amount that is needed to be reheated or thawed. This will also help with meal planning and make it easier to bring keto friendly foods to work or school for lunch.

You will also always have food ready to go if in a rush and have no time to cook.

A food scale can be a great tool when just starting out. You can be very surprised what an actual portion size looks like if you are trying to just "eye it." And when tracking macros to get into ketosis it is important to be accurate.

Keep some type of keto food ready made and on hand at all times. Whether it is fat bombs, cheese, cooked meat, or even leftovers. Having something ready to eat when you are starving and too tired to cook or don't have enough time will keep you from making a bad decision and eating non keto-friendly food. While this especially important when just starting out on the diet and your hunger hasn't decreased yet, you will find it can still be important even years into a ketogenic diet. You never know when something is going to come up or you are going to be too tired or even sick to be able to make yourself a meal. Do you really want to trust someone else with your ketosis? Always have food ready.

And if you can, remove all non keto approved carbohydrates from your kitchen. If you have other family members who are not ready or are unable to commit to a ketogenic lifestyle and have to keep the carbs around for them, put them all together in a cabinet by themselves that way you don't have to use that cabinet and you don't have to worry about craving them every time you see them.

Remember, the longer you remain on a ketogenic diet the easier it will be. Your taste buds will change over time and you will find yourself craving satiating, fatty meats instead of bread and French fries. You'll wonder how you ever found those high carb foods to be so appetizing. When you reach that point, you'll know you found your new way of life.

Chapter 9 - Maximize Your Fat Burning Potential

When it comes to maximizing the weight loss potential of the keto diet you may want to try combining it with the habit of intermittent fasting. The two types of weight loss both utilize the same bodily state, making them natural companions in your journey towards a happier and healthier you.

Most of us know what fasting means. It is the deliberate act of depriving oneself of food or drink for a set period of time. But that definition is not always accurate. There are different types of fasting that people may do. Some may fast for religious reasons while others may go on what can be considered as a partial fast.

You might find someone that does a juice fast where they only drink juice or water but does not eat. There is also a cleansing fast where one drinks water mixed with some simple sugars and cayenne pepper to clean the colon of toxins and food that may have built up.

For the most part, we all fast at some point every day. Generally, this is when we sleep. It is the period of time when we do not eat. Some people fast by skipping breakfast or dinner, others may choose to skip a meal here or there. There are all sorts of ways you can fast, but none of these are accurate enough to describe intermittent fasting.

The Basics of Intermittent Fasting

Intermittent fasting is when you choose to skip at least one meal during normal eating times. One could be considered fasting if they have not eaten anything for a period of eight hours or more.

As we discussed in Chapter 1, when you eat, the body immediately begins to break down the food and turn it into glucose. Glucose, in turn, starts the production of insulin and the insulin is used to aid the body in using the glucose for energy. It then stores any excess glucose as fat.

All of this happens with your regular diet. However, if you fast for 12 hours or more, the body's glucose levels will be depleted (since it can't really store it for the long term) and it will be forced to start burning the fat stores. This is the point when you begin to lose weight. It is also the ideal time to start exercising.

When you are fasting, there are no lists of foods you should or should not eat. The focus is more on when you should eat rather than what. So, you cannot consider intermittent fasting in the same way you would other types of diets but should view it more like an eating schedule.

There are several ways you can use intermittent fasting including:

- 16/8 fasts – where you fast for 16 hours and designate only 8 hours of the day to eat.
- Eat-Stop-Eat – where you fast for 24 hours only once or twice during the week. The rest of the days you follow your normal eating pattern.
- 5:2 – where you restrict your caloric intake to only 5-600 calories for 2 days out of the week but eat normally for the other 5 days. When you restrict your caloric intake in one of these methods, it should trigger weight loss and as long as you stick to your normal eating habits on the other days, you should find a nice healthy balance.

Most people have found success through one of the different methods of IF. The focus here is on forcing the body into a starvation mode so it begins to work at depleting its fat stores.

Basically, intermittent fasting is the act of eliminating food for a short period of time and then starting to consume again. Switching back and forth between fasting and eating is not the core of this effective approach. The key factor in its success is to ensure that when you eat, you are still making sure that you get all the nourishment you need when you are eating. This means taking in quality foods so that the body does not suffer from malnourishment. When planning your meals, make sure that you are supplying your body with the necessary macro and micronutrients and you can be relatively confident that the fasting approach will work.

<u>*How Insulin Plays a Role*</u>

Most of us have heard of insulin but may not really understand what it really is. Insulin is an essential hormone that aids in the distribution of nutrition throughout the body. When our insulin levels are high, the body is more likely to be in a storage mode. When it is low, our bodies look to the non-primary tissues for the fuel it needs.

Stress also plays a huge part in it as well. Everyone has some level of stress in their lives but some struggle with it more than others. You may not see it in your everyday practices, but evidence of stress is usually seen in those who have trouble sleeping, are restless, or have a constant feeling of tension.

These symptoms are a result of the body's release of the stress hormone, cortisol, which is responsible for the inborn "flight or fight" physiologic response. Cortisol can have an effect on your blood glucose levels.

When there is a prolonged period of cortisol stimulation, it will raise the blood glucose levels. When the adrenal glands release the cortisol, a message is sent throughout the body that more glucose is needed to prepare to face an impending threat. The liver responds to this message by triggering gluconeogenesis. In the life of our ancient ancestors, this surge of glucose was released when the decision was made to fight or flee from the threat, but in today's modern age, these extra energy stores mainly go unreleased, causing higher glucose and insulin levels in an attempt to bring it back down to normal.

This teaches us that even if we are consistent with our keto fast and do everything nutritionally to keep our blood glucose at bay; it is likely going to be stress that will have the biggest impact on our levels. So, a key factor in ensuring the success of the keto fast is to have a regular practice of reducing stress as a key part of keeping your blood glucose levels under control. Doing so with the only diet, may not be enough in some people. This is why some form of light cardio on fasting days and more rigorous exercise on the eating days may also be necessary.

In addition to exercise, others may also incorporate other stress-relieving activities into their normal routine. Studying or playing music, wearing eye shades while sleeping to block out light, earplugs to block out noise, watching television, taking walks, etc. There is a long list of stress relieving strategies you can apply to help you keep the body from producing too much blood glucose, so everything stays in balance.

The Impact of the Keto IF Diet on Insulin Levels

In order to achieve ketosis, the keto diet only allows you a very small amount of carbs from fruits and vegetables. This means that the consumption of any type of grain like pasta, refined sugars, dairy, corn, legumes, and rice is strictly off the table. Without these foods, your muscles and liver are forced to find alternative sources for their energy, primarily from your body's fat stores.

Once you understand the process, this starts to make sense. It is a logical means of controlling blood glucose levels. But there is one problem. The brain is designed to burn glucose and demands carbs for its energy source. When the levels are low, the brain will tell your liver to manufacture more ketones as a backup source of fuel.

The effectiveness of fasting depends a lot on how it's done. When you restrict the eating window to specific time periods many things can happen. There are two studies that showed that participants that ate normally one day and fasted the next day and continued on an alternate fasting program over a two-week period found that they did not all get the same results. One group showed improvement in their insulin sensitivity, but the second group showed no benefits whatsoever. In another study, the participants had a set eating window every day (restricting their eating to only two meals a day) showed significantly more improvement than the first study group.

This leads many people to wonder what caused the difference. It was clear that the results showed a fine line in how the keto fast could keep the insulin levels low and what happens when you starve the body. It was obvious that when fasting was taken to the extreme, it could be more harmful than good in the long run. Much of it depended on the individual's physical constitution as well as how they perceived and practiced fasting. A lot also had to do with how they were supplementing their meals and getting in those essential minerals and nutrients.

Insulin and Macronutrients

While the keto fast diet does not have any specific measurements that dictate what you are to eat or how much you are to eat, getting the right balance of macronutrients is essential. One person may be very diligent in making sure that they consume a significant quantity of macronutrients during their eating window, but another may not be so careful. These kinds of personal and individual decisions can drastically skew the results. For example, if you are fasting for 16 hours a day and eating from noon to 8 PM, your results will depend on what you are consuming. When you diligently ensure that you get enough of these macronutrients, you know that your body is getting a sufficient amount of energy even if you don't eat a lot during your eating window.

The reality is simple. Because high insulin levels is one of the key factors in developing insulin resistance, by following a dietary regimen that incorporates periods of time throughout the day where insulin is low, it becomes obvious that frequently eating will force the body to create more glucose, which in turn will force the body to try to control that glucose with insulin. So, if you want to keep insulin levels at bay, you need to keep glucose levels under control and the best way to do that is to have frequent periods of starvation. This calls into question the age-old belief that eating three meals a day is better for a balanced nutrition. Instead, it stands to reason that to control insulin, the opposite is true; we must eat fewer than three meals a day in order to deplete the body of blood glucose and keep insulin under control.

The Winning Combination

Another hormone that plays a critical part in our growth (especially during childhood) is the Insulin-like Growth Factor or the IGF-1. This is one of the most effective ways to activate those specific pathways that trigger cell growth and cell death in our bodies. The IGF-1 works in tandem with the HGH. When HGH is released into the bloodstream, the liver produces and releases IGF-1 at the same time. This automatically triggers a systemic growth in nearly all of the body's cells including bone, cartilage, kidney, lungs, muscles, nerves, and skin.

IGF-1 primary role is to promote cell growth. It holds in its power certain anti-aging and performance boosting effects, so you can build and retain muscle and bone mass even when you are fasting. It can affect the body in a similar way to insulin, lowering blood sugar, but not to the same extent.

IGF-1 and IGF-2 both are very similar to insulin in that they are mostly produced in the liver and are considered to be extensions of HGH creating the same basic effects on the body. Together they activate different receptors triggering growth in various cells in the body.

Everyone needs to have a moderate amount of IGF-1 in their bodies in order to maintain optimal health. However, too much or too little could raise your risk of mortality. So, it is very important to keep these hormones in balance.

The normal range of your IGF-1 varies depending on your age:

- Ages 0 to 3:   18-229 ng/mL
- Ages 4 to 8:   30-356 ng/mL

- Ages 8 to 13:   61-589 ng/mL
- Ages 14 to 22:   91-442 ng/mL
- Ages 23 to 35:   99-310 ng/mL
- Ages 36 to 50:   48-259 ng/mL
- Ages 51 to 65:   37-220 ng/mL
- Ages 66 to 80:   33-192 ng/mL
- Ages 81 to 91:   32-173 ng/mL

One way to keep your IGF-1 in check is by eating a diet that is low in sugar and processed carbohydrates. The more unprocessed and nutrient-dense foods you consume, the more they can help to encourage insulin sensitivity, which can better regulate your metabolism and increase the bio-activity of IGF-1.

In the end, having a balanced IGF-1 working with your insulin can be the ideal way to establish an anabolic state in the body and give your immune system the support it needs to keep you healthy while you're on your KETO Fast.

Body Composition

The most important hormone when it comes to keeping up and improving your body composition is insulin. If your insulin levels are always in an elevated state, then no matter what you do, your body won't be able to burn your fat stores and will shift into a storage mode. Therefore, it is necessary to keep your insulin levels as low as possible. Eating a high-carb diet several times a day will counteract any nutritional advances you may be hoping to make.

Remember, insulin only rises when your blood sugar levels rise as a means of counteracting the spikes, which are most often caused by a high-carb diet. The secret to getting rid of that excess body fat is to keep insulin levels low and drastically cut back on your carbs.

Developing the skill to burn fat is very much like learning to master an art. It's all about balance. When your glucose levels finally run out, your body will automatically make the switch and in time, you will enter that all-important state of ketosis. The keto fast diet can speed up this process and keep you in a fat burning state for a longer period of time. When you are in ketosis, you will then be using your fat cells as a fuel source, and you will start to see the pounds begin to melt away.

Keep in mind that while the calories in and out are keys to energy balance, a more important element to control when you're trying to lose weight is the hormonal balance in your body. Since insulin is the primary hormone in maintaining a healthy balance and body composition, you want to keep it down for the majority of the time, which can be done through keto fasting.

How to Get Started

Now it is time to get down to the real nitty-gritty of keto fasting. To start with, it doesn't really matter which eating window you choose but to get the most out of the process, most would suggest that you skip your early morning breakfast and have it in the afternoon. This will put you into an underfed state for the better part of the day. Your first meal of the day should actually be low in calories so that you leave the table still feeling a little hungry.

First, you must understand when the fasting period officially starts. Surprisingly, it is not when you finish that last morsel of food at the end of your eating window. Even though you will no longer be eating anything else, the nutrients in the food are still going to have to go through the digestive process so that the body can absorb them. Depending on how much food you consume, expect that your body does not enter the fasting state until around 4-6 hours after your last bite. This time period can vary from person to person and depending on the contents of your last meal. So, for simplicity sake, start counting your fasting time at least 30 minutes after your last meal. For some, this time period will be longer but it should not be shorter than this.

Keep in mind that carbohydrates are the culprit. If your meal has a significant amount of carbs, your insulin levels will be high and your blood glucose levels as well. They will remain high for a longer period of time, which will delay the amount of time it will take for your body to go into ketosis. If you're on the ketogenic diet though, then your body will go into ketosis much faster and hopefully, you will be in a ketogenic state when you finally go to sleep. By the time you rise in the morning, your body will be primed towards burning fat to get you through the day.

Sleep is Hugely Important

It is important that you give serious consideration to your sleep because it is directly related to achieving ketosis as well as maintaining your overall health. When neglected, our bodies do not go through a complete repairing cycle. It is during sleep that your body releases HGH so without it, or when you don't get enough of it, your general condition of health will suffer.

You need to get around 7-8 hours of sleep every night; anything less automatically puts your body under stress, which will put you in an insulin resistant state, your glucose levels will be too high, and you won't have enough energy to get you through the day. As a result, you'll begin to lose muscle and all the fat will go into the fat stores.

But in today's modern world where we have such busy lives, it is hard to get a full 8 hours of sleep a night. You might feel this is an impossible task, but if you start paying closer attention to your body's circadian rhythm, you might find that your problem is that you're trying to sleep at the wrong time. For most people, the optimum sleep time is between 10 PM and 6 AM but that does not apply to all people. Some are morning people and others are night owls, and of course, there are a whole bunch of variations in between. Where you are will depend on your personal circadian rhythm or your internal 24-hour clock that regulates the periods when you are most alert and the best time to eat or sleep. So, while the general recommendation is the 10-6 sleep timeframe, there is no such thing as one size fits all. You need to match your activities with your natural internal rhythm, so you can get the right amount of sleep on a regular basis.

You can start by paying close attention to your body. Your circadian rhythm is a combination of physiological, mental, and behavioral patterns played out throughout the day. Before the advent of the sundial, people managed to get up and go through life without an external device telling them when to do anything. There was no such thing as an alarm clock or a bedtime. They lived by the cues they received from the environment. They got up with the sun and went to sleep when it was dark. The climate could also have played a role in when to get up and go to sleep.

Your circadian rhythm influences more than when you sleep and wake up. It also tells the body when to release hormones, adjust its temperature and perform other bodily functions. These rhythms are not consistent throughout life; as you get older your body will naturally adjust to certain changes. You should notice that when the body is exposed to light, the brain will send a signal to raise the temperature and produce the hormone cortisol. This supplies energy to rouse you and start the day. The opposite is true for when darkness falls; the brain's signal is sent to produce melatonin, the hormone that helps us to sleep. If you have a healthy sleep pattern, then your melatonin levels will remain high throughout the night until the body is once again exposed to light.

As we age, the amount of melatonin in our bodies begins to gradually decrease so we start waking up earlier in the day. This change starts in our thirties and will continue to decrease throughout the remainder of our lives. One study showed that we naturally start waking up earlier and earlier as we age. In our twenties, it is easy to stay in bed until 9:30 or later, but by the time we are in our thirties, we are naturally waking up at around 8:00; in our forties it is 7:30, and in our fifties we are aroused by 7:00, and by the time we are in our sixties it is difficult to stay in bed past 6:30 in the morning. It is therefore important to understand when our bodies are telling us to sleep so we can get to bed at the right time.

Work also influences how much time we have to sleep too. Depending on when you wake up, the best time to start work is between 2½ to 3 hours after you get up. That gives our bodies enough time to shake off the grogginess and build up alertness. For younger people, that could be sometime around noon and for older people that could be much earlier. Unfortunately, this type of schedule is not often accepted in our modern society that demands a constant flow of work, which sadly is achieved by robbing us of our much-needed sleep.

Exercise

With the keto fast diet, you need to put in some exercise in order to get the best bang for your buck. The optimum time for a good workout is usually around 4 hours before retiring for the evening. That is usually the point when we are at our peak in terms of strength, and lung function. So, based on what time dictates for you go to bed, you can schedule your exercise routine in at that point.

Once you learn how to read your body, it will be easy to find out the optimum time for you to incorporate all the facets of the keto fast diet into your daily routine. By matching it up based on your natural body rhythms and not by a specific clock, you will be more likely to achieve success and feel good about it at the same time.

Another way you can ensure better sleep is to block out any exposure you have to blue light. This is not the natural sunlight streaming through your windows in the mornings but is the kind of light that emits from your devices and gadgets. Even with your eyes closed; this light causes your subconscious mind to suppress the production of melatonin, which will cause you to wake up much earlier than you would naturally. If you are in an environment with a lot of blue light, try wearing blue light blocking glasses when you go to sleep, and chances are you'll sleep all through the night.

Without adequate sleep, your body will struggle to reach ketosis, and you will not achieve the kind of results you are trying to get.

Understanding Your Metabolism

It is important to know the steps for getting started on a keto fast. Your goal is to get your body's metabolism to make the switch from burning glucose to burning fat and all of that starts in your stomach.

The stomach is the part of our body that is most sensitive to external influences. Everything you swallow, from a single stick of gum to our favorite foods will end up inside our intestines where the whole process begins. From the moment you make your first swallow, the stomach will begin to release hydrochloric acid to start the digestive process.

Your intestines are crawling with millions of tiny bacteria or tiny microorganisms that are sending out messages to the rest of the body about what should be done at any point in time. If your stomach is not healthy, you might experience brain fog, sluggishness, and even joint pain. Believe it or not, all of these microorganisms are in control of our appetite, hormones, metabolism, and even our mood. Above all else, keeping good healthy food in our bodies is the single most important secret to living a healthy and productive life. You need to fuel all of that by putting the proper foods into your body.

- Dark leafy greens - provide fiber, vitamins, enzymes, and minerals.
- Fat and protein - help the digestive system.
- Fermented foods - add healthy bacteria to your gut. Good sources of fermented foods are sauerkraut, kimchi, pickles, raw yogurt, kefir, and tempeh.

You can make many fermented foods at home if you have the time. Store bought fermented foods are not nearly as effective as a pure homemade brand and you may find that you're getting more sugar in your system than you want.

To kick-start your metabolism in the right way, you need to pay close attention to your inflammation levels. Gauge how you feel after eating something. If you find that you are feeling sluggish or are having a higher degree of pain in your joints, chances are your body is rejecting that food and you probably should cut it from your diet.

As you go through your new diet, you will have to pay close attention to how your body responds to everything you eat. But in addition, you may have to take another more drastic approach to protect your internal systems.

1. Do a pantry sweep.

    Go through your pantry and get rid of everything that is heavy in carbohydrates. This includes bread, cereals, fruit, pasta, potatoes, rice, sugar, etc. If they are not in your house, you won't be tempted to eat them. Stock your pantry full of keto rich foods to keep you from being pulled in the direction of carbohydrates.

2. Stock up on keto staples.

    These include:

    a) Extra virgin olive oil

    b) Extra virgin coconut oil

    c) Organic Ghee

    d) Frozen vegetables

    e) Frozen Meat

f) Pink Himalayan Rock Salt

g) Turmeric

h) Ginger

i) Cinnamon

If you do this from the beginning, every time you open your cabinet, you know you are getting something that is nutritious on the ketogenic diet. You won't have to read labels, count calories, or figure out fat grams.

Finally, take some time to figure out your macronutrients. Especially in the very beginning stages of the keto fast, pay close attention to how many macros you are getting in each meal. This may mean weighing your food to make sure that everything you eat is within the ketogenic macronutrient rations as follows:

- Carbohydrates from vegetables and meats should be somewhere between 30-50 grams per day maximum. The lower your carbs the sooner you will achieve ketosis.

- Proteins should be moderate with around 15-25% total calories of protein consumed each day. If you are a sedentary person, then you should adjust that percentage downward for best effect. A general guideline to follow is a minimum of 07 to 1.3 grams for each pound of lean body mass you have.

- Fat should make up the rest of your meal plan with more than 70-80%. Keep in mind that fat can be an extreme source of dense calories so even though there is no limit on how much you can consume if you're trying to lose weight, eating too much of it can be counter-productive.

<u>*When Can You Go Back to Carbs*</u>

Getting started on a ketogenic fast doesn't have to be complicated, but we live in a world full of foods that are working contrary to your goals. Almost everything we eat is loaded with carbohydrates, trans fats, and sugars. Still, if you are determined to go low-carb, you need to be realistic about what is really causing your health problems.

Our lives are much too complex to blame everything wrong with us on carbohydrates. It is usually a combination of factors and carbohydrates are just one single part of it. As we have already discussed our poor health and weight problems could also be the result of too much stress, a lack of adequate sleep, or our environment.

While reaching a state of ketosis can alleviate many of our physical ailments, don't assume it is the miracle that will give you back your youth and deliver you to perfect health all on its own. Even if you are in ketosis, you don't need to stay in ketosis for the duration.

It will take time for you to reach a state of ketosis (up to two weeks) and the longer you can maintain that state the better your results will be. However, once your body develops a good fat-adaptation, consistently maintaining a state of ketosis won't always be necessary.

At some point, you won't need to or even want to maintain the keto fast and you can switch out of it. Some people will want to go off the program during holidays or special events, others may choose to boost their athletic ability and will need their bodies to produce more glycogen, and others may choose to try an alternative diet for some other reason. Whatever the case, being able to transition from the ketogenic diet will be necessary. If you do, expect that moving out of a state of ketosis can bring some surprising results:

- You will gain weight.

  Almost immediately your body will put on weight. This is because when you stopped eating carbs the body was forced to burn up all its glucose and excess water. So, you started losing the water weight you had been retaining for so long. When you begin consuming carbs again, that water will return.

  This has absolutely nothing to do with your state of ketosis but is simply the body's natural reaction to the nutrients found in carbs. The same is true when you have a high sodium intake; your body will naturally hold onto more water. So, when you are on keto, your body will maintain less glycogen and you will see the changes when you go off.

- Gradually go off keto.

Don't make a sudden change to your old eating habits. For the first week, try to consume only small amounts of carbohydrates in the form of tubers and vegetables. Eat more carrots, beets, and berries. Continue to eat the low-carb vegetables because you will benefit from their micronutrients and anti-cancerous agents, but stay away from starchy foods for now.

- Gradually start to add starch in the second week.

In the second week, you can start adding potatoes or rice for your meals but only on those days when you are more physically active. Keep it to smaller amounts so you can stay in semi-ketosis for at least a portion of the day. Keep your carb intake at this point to between 100-200 grams.

- Add more in the third week.

By the third week, you can eat more of the starchy carbs like fruits and grains but try to boost up your physical activity at the same time. At this point, you will be off keto so to maintain your improved health; you need to focus on controlling your insulin. By this time, your insulin sensitivity should have seen some improvement but the question as to how much carbs you can take without destroying all of your efforts will depend on how lean you are and how much muscle mass you have achieved. Try not to go above 300 grams per day as a maximum.

- Keep the fasting going.

  As long as you keep the momentum going with your fasting periods you should be able to keep your fat-burning status in check. Don't go all the way back to your old habits by eating more meals a day. By keeping the fasting routine, even if you do go back to carbs, you will remain in a state where you are burning fat.

- Continue your workouts.

  If you're going to go back to carbs, the best time to consume them is after a workout. This is the point where your muscle glycogen stores have been depleted and the body needs that extra fuel.

- Eat carbs with care.

  When you introduce carbs back into your diet, there should be a method to your madness. Your first meal for each day, when you literally break your fast, should still have a very low glycemic count. By doing this, you will keep your fat burning efforts closer to a fasted state for longer.

If you find that you like the benefits of the ketogenic diet, but you still want the pleasures of having some carbs from time to time, you might want to consider trying a Cyclical Ketogenic

Diet. This is a system where you do keto for a set period of time and then switch back to carbs, and then repeat.

What is so great about this method is that it can be structured to your liking. When you go back on carbs (called refeeds), you can choose to do it once a week or once a month, or even occasionally when you are with friends. By combining this with your keto fast, you never have to concern yourself with missing out on any of your favorite foods.

Ideally, when you practice this method, you want to ease into the refeeding. You will find that once you get your keto fast going in full swing, it won't be so easy to go back full force to your old eating habits. The first time, limit yourself to only high glycemic carbohydrates and then the next time, eat only low glycemic.

Stay on the refeed for one or two days then the rest of the week stay on your keto fast. Here is a sample schedule you might want to practice.

- Stay on your keto fast until you are fully adapted to the new eating style. This will take about 2-3 weeks.
- Schedule your refeed on a day when you are most physically active.

- While fasting, make sure your workout is more intense, so you deplete your glycogen stores and your muscles are more in need of carbs.
- Try to include some High-Intensity-Intermittent-Training.
- After the workout, eat your high glycemic carbs (rice, potatoes, bananas, etc.) This will cause your insulin level to spike.
- Allow your insulin to rise but for the rest of the eating window, continue to eat your carbs along with a moderate amount of protein (lean meats) and limit your fats as your body will store them if your insulin is too high.

Of course, like with any other diet, you must take extra care when you break your cycle as your body will react differently. It is not recommended that you practice this on a regular basis since doing so can disrupt the rhythm you've worked so hard to develop. Don't stay off your cycle more than one or two days or you might find that you have to start the whole process over from scratch to continue with your weight loss.

Getting Your Body Adjusted to Fasting

Fasting is not always easy. You have been eating the same way for a long time and it will be difficult in the beginning to readjust to this new method. You will have to do more than change the times you eat and what you eat. It doesn't hurt to have a little bit of help in making that adjustment so here are a few basic guidelines that can smooth the way for you to incorporate this new way of life into your regular routine.

Start by Getting Rid of the Carbs

Start with a simple low carb diet. If you are accustomed to eating a lot of carbs every day then you won't be able to start the fasting phase right away. Instead, start by cutting down the number of carbs you consume and give your body time to make the adjustment.

Once you're better adjusted to cutting back on your carbs, then start with the ketogenic diet and maintain that for 2-3 weeks. At this point, you can gradually start narrowing down your eating window. Many newbies consider skipping breakfast and eating only lunch and dinner but remember to follow your circadian rhythm.

On a ketogenic diet, try to get a nice balance of food:

- 70% fat

- 20% protein

- 10% carbohydrates

When you do start eating again, your first meal should always be with low glycemic foods that don't have a high caloric count. This could be 3-4 eggs, some spinach, a little butter and some nuts (around 500 calories).

Increase Your Fasting Period

After a few weeks on the ketogenic diet, your body should have gone into a state of ketosis. As long as you keep your carbohydrates below your daily 10% allowance, your glycogen stores should be depleted. This is a good time to measure your ketones. If you have a high blood ketone level and a low blood glucose level, then you are in ketosis.

This is when you should start putting more emphasis on the fasting phase. Longer faster periods can now be introduced, which will speed up your progress. If you're feeling more adventurous, you could try a 24-hour fast or try a 20/4 (The Warrior) fast but if you're still adjusting then try to keep your fasting near the 16/8 mark.

Notch It up a Bit

After you've gotten used to the 16/8 fast and have a couple of 24-hour fasts under your belt, you can start experimenting with more extreme fasting times. Some try to do 40-48 hour fasts or 5-day fasts, but these are difficult to accomplish. While it is possible to do this on a physical level, it is probably more psychologically demanding for most people.

Rather than take such drastic measures, try fasting for as long as you can. If you start to feel pain or any other type of discomfort, there is nothing wrong with going back to your 16/8 or the fasting periods you have become accustomed to.

While this step is not necessary, it can be quite a morale booster to see exactly how much your body can withstand. For most people, the most difficult part is getting past the 24-hour part, once you cross that line your body will pretty much be able to handle just about anything you throw at it. Remember, it is not the length of the fast that makes it hard, it is finding ways to keep your blood sugar stable during that time.

If you begin to feel symptoms like fatigue or overall discomfort during longer fasts, then consider boosting the amount of sodium in your diet. Anything like lethargy, muscle cramps, and hypoglycemia, these are not so much from what you are not eating but instead from an imbalance of electrolytes in your body, and not from starvation. When you feel that happening, you could try to take a rest but if the feeling continues, then you should stop your fast.

Conclusion

You have learned that the ketogenic diet has been around for decades, it was founded by doctors as a safe and healthy way to manage many neurological disorders and allow many to live symptom free lives. By training your body to run in a natural state of ketosis you are automatically burning your fat stores while eating a variety of foods and never having to feel hungry. If you choose to take it a step further and include the 16/8 intermittent fasting method with this diet you will find an even greater increase of fat burned throughout the day, causing you to lose even more weight, faster.

There are many foods to choose from on a ketogenic diet including many desserts. There is no need to count calories because eating such high fat foods helps to keep you feeling full longer, naturally lessening the amount of calories you consume on a daily basis. It is even recommended to eat high fat sweets and fat bombs to help keep your body burning fat for energy. You don't even have to turn down your friends parties or stay behind when everyone goes out to eat or to celebrate. There are many options while dining out and you can even have the occasional alcoholic drink after fat adapted. Once you get through adaptation, you won't believe the new found energy you have and the amazing and delicious choices of food.

I'm sure that by this time you are sick of having to explain to your friends repeatedly what you have been doing to lose so much weight, please let them know how great the ketogenic diet is working for you and recommend this book to help get them started too.

Thank you for downloading this book and I hope that you found it informative. I wish you the best of luck on your new weight loss journey with the ketogenic diet.

www.ingramcontent.com/pod-product-compliance
Lightning Source LLC
Chambersburg PA
CBHW061807250726

48657CB00001B/322